Guide to
Winning Mind Games

Keep Your Hair and Your Health

Manuel Antonio Lopez

iUniverse LLC
Bloomington

WINNING MIND GAMES
KEEP YOUR HAIR AND YOUR HEALTH

iUniverse books may be ordered through booksellers or by contacting:

iUniverse
1663 Liberty Drive
Bloomington, IN 47403
www.iuniverse.com
1-800-Authors (1-800-288-4677)

ISBN: 978-1-4917-1910-7 (sc)
ISBN: 978-1-4917-1911-4 (hc)
ISBN: 978-1-4917-1912-1 (e)

Library of Congress Control Number: 2013923530

Printed in the United States of America.

iUniverse rev. date: 1/16/2014

Acknowledgments
This book would not have been possible without the
support of my wife and two sons

Photo Credits
Photographs by the author, Pablo Lopez,
Diego Lopez, and Carol Peredo Lopez

Graphics
Pablo Lopez

Contents

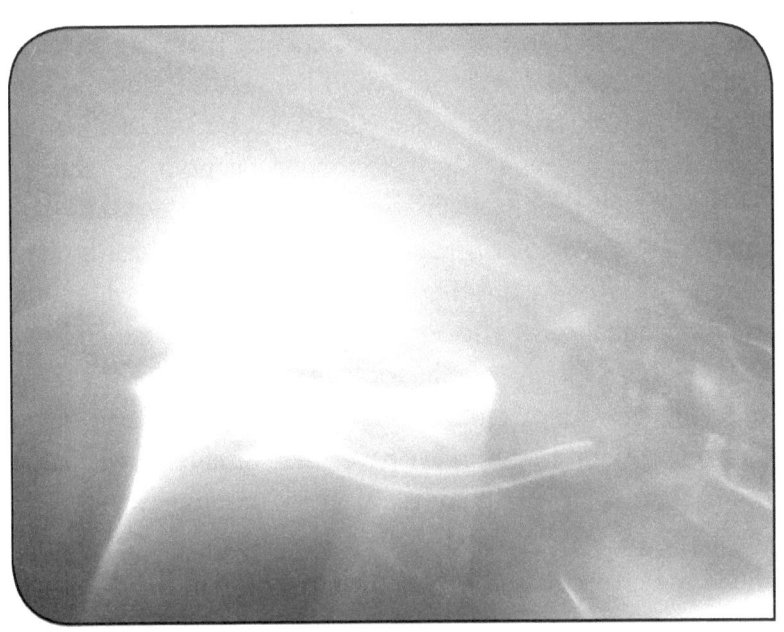

Introduction

This book provides engineering solutions to problems based on my own experiences and human behavioral data that I collected over the past thirty-eight years. Even though most of this data is based on observations of changes in the behaviors of a man, most of these elements would also apply to a woman. The basic principle, hidden in the context throughout this book, is based on creating an analogy between engineering system standards and the human "machine" in order to analyze and solve human problems.

This book discusses and demonstrates how to transform one's state of mind from adapted hyperactive—being "stressed out"—to relaxed. This book is based on my personal journey of experiencing and overcoming these changes. I discuss my three-year transformation experience from an adapted hyperactive stressed state of mind, where I was losing my hair at an excessively fast rate and gaining weight, to a transformed relaxed state of mind. My hair stopped falling and I started growing thick healthy hair, and I also lost the weight I had gained. I learned to control my stress, keep my healthy hair and maintain my weight thereafter. Since everyone is different, each individual must choose how to apply these experiences to his or her journey. I undertook a three-year journey from enduring an undetectable adapted hyperactive state to being at a relaxed state of mind. I have successfully stayed in the latter state for over thirty-eight years. Having experienced both the hyperactive and relaxed states has allowed me to make comparisons and observations of human behavior and physical changes.

It has been a progressive and deliberate experiment. I have avoided all types of external media influence over the last thirty-eight years and have noted changes based on the environment, changes in personal behavior, and the effects these changes have on the human electromechanical body, unpredicted mutations, mental health, and values. I have also observed the transmission of these changes across genes.

This book states observations and methods to disprove or confirm my theories about what causes the onset of hyperactivity, the side effects, and what it takes to reverse a hyperactive state of mind. This book defines terms such as *stress* as a hyperactive condition and defines a relaxed state of mind as a peaceful one that counters stress. It explains how diseases are associated with the onset of hyperactivity, their side effects, and the permanent physical changes they instigate. It also discusses how to use meditation to reverse a hyperactive condition. This book uncovers fresh information that leads to new antidotes, new discoveries, and a better life.

This book may seem a little difficult to understand at first since the changes described are different from the normal way of life as we know it. This book will need to be read again and again; as an individual evolves or changes from one state of mind to another, the reading will start to make sense and the words will reveal their true meaning. In other words, as the mind and body begin to slow down, one will see life from a different medium, a relaxed mind and body, and will see things differently for a better life.

Manuel A. Lopez is a professional engineer. He is an expert in configuration control systems and how dynamics and systems go together. He has over thirty-eight years of experience in analyzing mechanical and electrical systems and how they interact with human behavior. He consolidates and assimilates through processes in software systems.

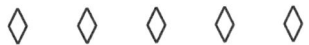

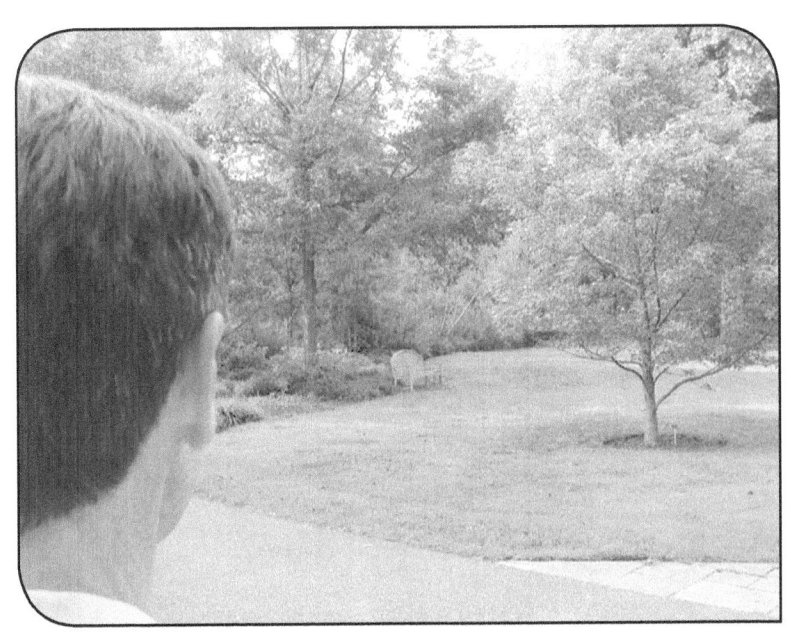

Chapter 1
Adapted Hyperactive State (AHS) Theory

Adapted Hyperactive State (AHS)

AHS is an adapted accelerated or hyperactive condition, which happens when both mind and body adapt or memorize an accelerated or hyperactive condition, which results in a permanent chronic or nervous state of the mind and body. The lifestyle changes and things look different when an individual is moving at a faster pace; values are impacted, material gratification is necessary, senses are exaggerated, sexual gratification is required, and satisfaction is constantly needed to cope with stress. Desires increase, as does the appetite for food. The need for food is exaggerated and triggered more often.

Hunger can strike as often as every fifteen minutes after having a full meal and can reoccur throughout the day. Food is continuously ingested to satisfy hunger, which causes mental or stomach pain. This uncontrollable hyperactive state of the mind is constantly active or turned on, day and night. While an individual is sleeping or trying to relax, the body is still processing enormous amounts of food, thus producing excessive energy and sweat to cool it down.

Adapted Hyperactivity or Staying On

Repetitive instances of nervous activity can cause the nervous triggers to stay on permanently. This nervous condition causes the body's organs to mutate or adapt to support this new energy demand. This means that the increased energy requirements stay on, while an individual is relaxing, working, sleeping, reading, and eating. This permanent condition is not easily apparent or visible. It becomes the new way of life.

Repetition

Repetitive nervous activity can cause the nervous trigger to stay on permanently. This means that the nervous system does not go back to the relaxed state; therefore, the nervous system is permanently active. The body organs can adapt and mutate to support the accelerated condition. This change can occur over a short time—in as little as six months—when the body is exposed to this repetitive use of the nervous trigger.

Why Does It Appear Natural?

AHS is an adapted hyperactive condition that appears natural or normal to the human body, especially if an individual has had this condition for a long time and if he or she has learned to live with it. A condition is considered natural only if the change is one that everyone experiences. For example, baldness appears natural if the majority of men are shown to experience the condition.

AHS Changes Based on Age—Main Causes

AHS can happen to anyone regardless of age. Age is not a factor here; both young and old are vulnerable to the same side effects. Men from twenty-one through sixty-five years of age are the most vulnerable to adapting to AHS. The critical age for a man is forty; this is when he starts to slow down and exercises less. Exercise can play a positive role in reversing AHS if performed along with meditation techniques.

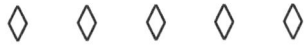

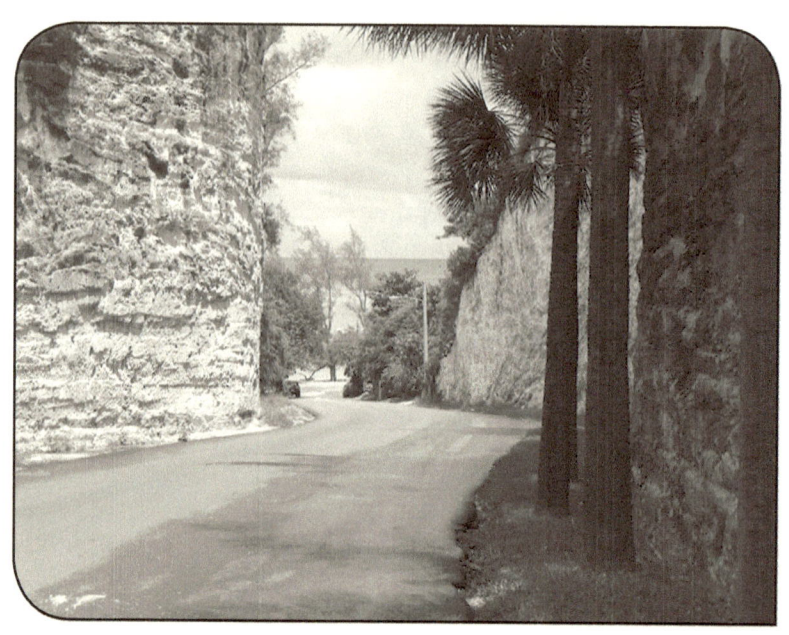

Chapter 2
The Nervous System Theory

Explaining the Nervous System

The nervous system is an uncontrollable mechanism that turns on and off during panic or in response to a stressful situation. There are two mental states: one is the normal or relaxed state, and the other is the hyperactive or nervous state. In the relaxed state, the body's system is operating at a slower and more controlled nervous frequency, where most of the actions happen after they are commanded by the mind. In the hyperactive or nervous state, the body's system is operating at a higher nervous frequency with little or no mind control. Actions are driven by the nervous system, and the mind control follows to correct the action taken or the situation. In other words, the nervous system automatically controls actions, speed, and body movements based on learned commands.

Nervous Trigger

The nervous system can be unconsciously turned on by external influences. For example, if an individual is exposed to a panic-inducing situation, the brain triggers the nervous system and releases an extreme rush of adrenaline so that the person is able to automatically and quickly react to protect or defend him- or herself from danger. The brain's nervous trigger can automatically turn itself on during routine, everyday situations, such as trying to meet deadlines, driving, receiving disagreeable news, experiencing emotions, and working in a fast-paced environment.

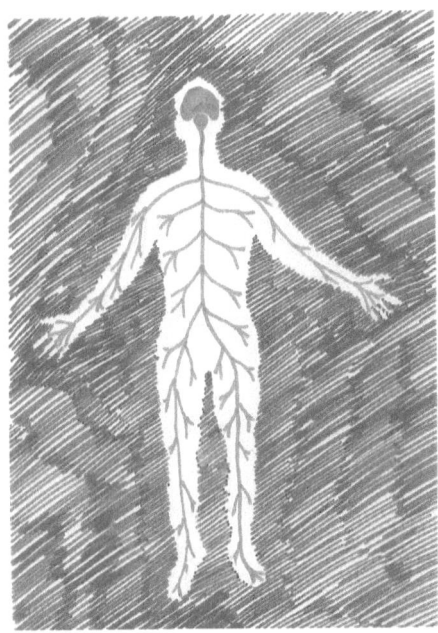

Hyperactive
Nervous System

The brain's two operating frequencies can coexist side by side; one is the slow, normal, everyday relaxed and controlled frequency, and the other is the fast, nervous, and uncontrollable frequency, which turns on during a panic-inducing or emergency situation. People can learn to control both frequencies and be able to turn the nervous frequency on and off at will when needed. People can learn to identify the relaxed and nervous frequency states and know when they are functioning at one or the other. This learned control allows people to benefit from the nervous energy to perform demanding tasks and at the same time benefit from the ability to be in the relaxed condition, which allows the body to truly relax and recharge. I do not recommend turning on the nervous system for any longer than two weeks, since at this time, the body organs start to permanently adapt to the new state.

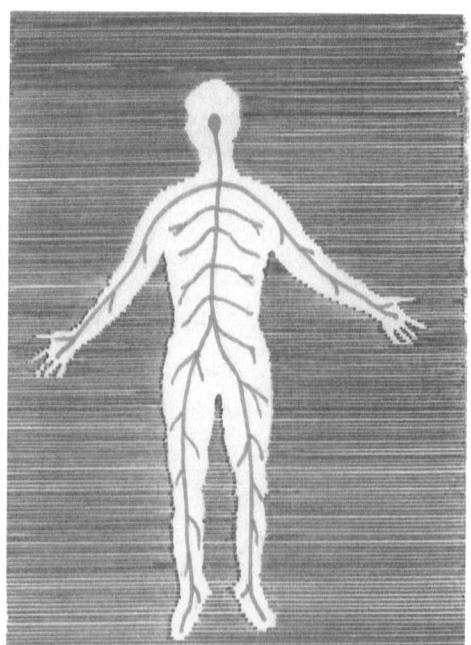

Relaxed Nervous System

The brain's nervous trigger can easily be turned on, but it can be very difficult to turn off, depending on the person's state of mind and how long it has stayed on. Turning it off can take hours, days, weeks, or months, or it may stay on permanently, depending on how long it has stayed on.

The nervous system trigger is directly related to the unique level of sensitivity of the individual, which directly affects how his or her body responds to external motivators, such as infections, temperatures, bacteria, allergies, and pain.

The greater the nervous sensitivity, the greater the effect it has on the body. A relaxed individual exposed to a hot object has less of a reaction to pain than a nervous individual.

Keeping a nervous system turned on weakens the immune system, leaving the individual vulnerable to bacteria or germs when compared to a healthy, relaxed individual.

Unstoppable Nervous System

A nervous mental condition can be learned; unfortunately, it can also harm the body. A nervous condition, once learned, is difficult to reverse since it affects or changes many of the body systems linked to and operated by the brain. Once the nervous trigger has been on for a long time, it tends to stay on. The longer it has stayed on, the longer it takes to reverse this condition.

The accelerated condition increases the mind-control frequency and stores new memories of all new learned body functions and behaviors at this higher operating frequency. Stored memories of body functions, such as walking, running, playing sports, talking, sleeping, thinking, and remembering are saved at this higher frequency. It takes more effort to reverse all these learned abilities back to the normal slower frequency than to adapt to the higher AHS frequency. The older the individual, the longer it takes to reverse the process, but it can be done; success depends on the individual's ability to learn and adapt.

This reversal process must be performed gradually in order to allow time for the mind and body to establish or reestablish communications at a slower frequency. This is the basis for the reversal theory.

Why Does the Nervous System Turn On?

The nervous system turns on in order to keep up with fast-paced activities, such as in media or games or a high-stress working environment. If the nervous system does not turn on, the mind cannot keep up with most of the scenes of fast-moving media, play fast games, or keep up with the pace of a higher-stress work environment and is unable to keep up with fast-moving everyday activities.

The mind learns by doing; therefore, the nervous sensitivity can be reversed, controlled, or conditioned to be less responsive. The mind can learn to be less sensitive to touch, smell, vision, taste, and hearing. It can even condition the body to move slowly or be less sensitive to touch or even learn to walk on hot surfaces.

Analog versus Digital

Analog versus Digital Signals

Comparing AHS versus non-AHS is like comparing digital movement (AHS) to analog movement (non-AHS). Move like an analog system rather than like a digital system in order to learn to control the nervous system. An analog signal moves slowly and gradually from low to high, while digital signals are either on or off instantly. A digital signal changes suddenly from a zero-gain signal to a 100 percent gain signal instantly; this is referred to as a step chart.

Muscle Frequency Based on Mass

Eye Movement
The eye is the primary conduit through which external motivating frequencies make their way into an individual's nervous system. Adaptation to AHS results in a condition that causes excessive and uncontrollable or rapid eye movements and blinking of the eyelids, which is required to mitigate the burning sensation from overly sensitive eyes.

Muscle Movement
The smaller the muscle, the less mass it has and the quicker it can keep up with the AHS frequency. Bigger muscle groups cannot move to a high frequency. Therefore, learning to control movements of the smaller muscle groups is important in controlling AHS. Learning to control smaller muscle groups so that they move only when commanded is one way to monitor and control AHS.

Changes to the Nervous System

AHS changes the nervous system. The nervous system becomes hypersensitive; with less mental control, more gratification and pleasures are needed more frequently to relieve stress; the body becomes more sensitive to pain and to external factors, such as airborne elements or heat.

AHS Changes Based on Size and Body Constitution

The smaller the body size, the more vulnerable the body is to adapting to AHS. This is because the lower the muscle mass, the less effort is needed to move muscles to a higher AHS frequency. A smaller individual can move faster than a larger individual. AHS has to do with the ability of the body's smaller muscle groups to reach the frequency of the body's nervous energy for a period long enough for the body to adapt. Therefore, the smaller muscle groups, such as the eye muscles and muscles of the eyelids and fingers are prone to acquiring and adapting AHS from higher external frequencies. Individuals who are larger in size will be more resistant to acquiring AHS.

Power of the Human Machine

The human machine can learn by doing; it can adapt, get stronger, and become tireless at will. The body can be taught to slow down or control the hyperactive nervous state and to regain the long-lost happiness, friendship, and values and to help rediscover a new and a renewed individual.

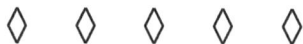

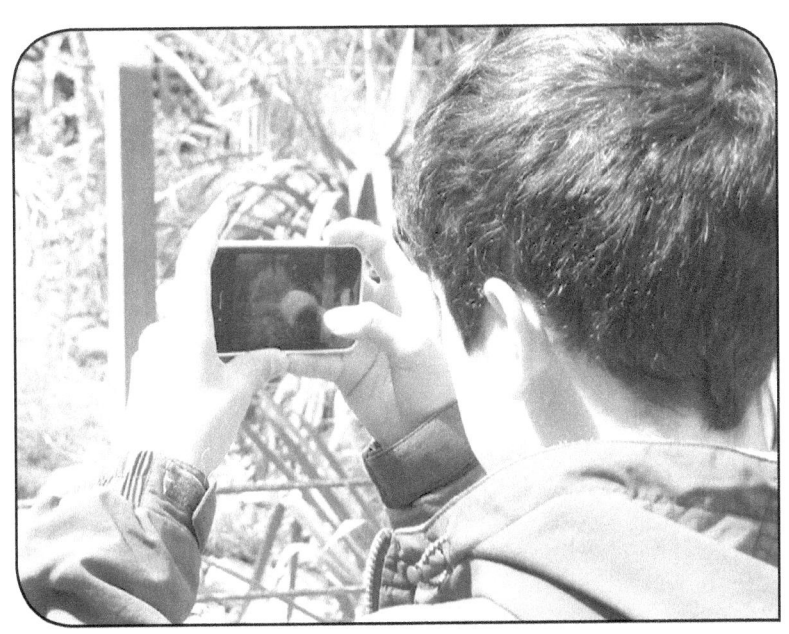

Chapter 3
Unconscious Learned Behavior Theory

Unconscious Learned Behavior

The mind learns by doing even if the individual is not aware of this unconscious process. The individual is aware of what he is doing but he is not aware that he has an unconscious process. The mind can learn to dislike, to socialize, to be shy, or to be aggressive; it can learn hyperactivity, a game, a desire, or stress. It can learn to be overweight and can learn to be outgoing. The mind can learn these conditions unconsciously if exposed to them long enough.

Changes in behavior can be learned in as little as six months to a year if one is exposed to the conditions daily or in less time if one is exposed to them continuously or twenty-four hours a day. Unfortunately, some of these learned conditions can cause harm to the mind and body or cause the body to prematurely mutate.

Permanent Changes

Behavior can be learned in as little as six months to a year. The body adapts to or memorizes a particular nervous state of mind when exposed to an accelerated condition for a long period of time. The metabolism changes and adapts to support the new mental condition and stays permanently in that state.

The new nervous state of mind is gratifying until the side effects start to surface or reveal themselves. Some individuals can cope better than others with this change in mental state, depending on their body composition, when in their lives this change occurred, and whether the change occurred gradually or quickly, or it may depend on other factors, such as the extent of exposure to an accelerated environment or the person's mental health.

Mutation

AHS can lead to premature body mutation in as little as six months to a year. A human body can adapt and mutate faster than ever imagined. It no longer takes millions of years for the body to mutate; this principle violates the laws of evolution.

Initial Consequences of AHS

Adaptation to AHS leads to side effects. The initial side effects can be seen in an increase in appetite, impatience, lack of sleep, circles around the eyes, some hair loss, dandruff, itchiness of the scalp, weight gain, rapid eye movement, excessive blinking, lack of concentration, uncontrollable urge, nervous energy, continuously upset stomach, clumsiness or bumping into things, speech errors, a fast laugh, and hyperactivity.

What Happens When the Nervous System Turns On?

The relevant part of the nervous system is technically referred to as the autonomic system. It is located at the center of the brain or on the upper part of the spinal cord. When turned on, it starts to generate excessive internal heat. This heat is generally released through the upper part of the brain and in turn makes the brain hot. This excessive heat can be seen since it leads to excessive perspiration at the scalp. This nervous activity can unconsciously turn on when the brain or the mind loses control of the nervous system.

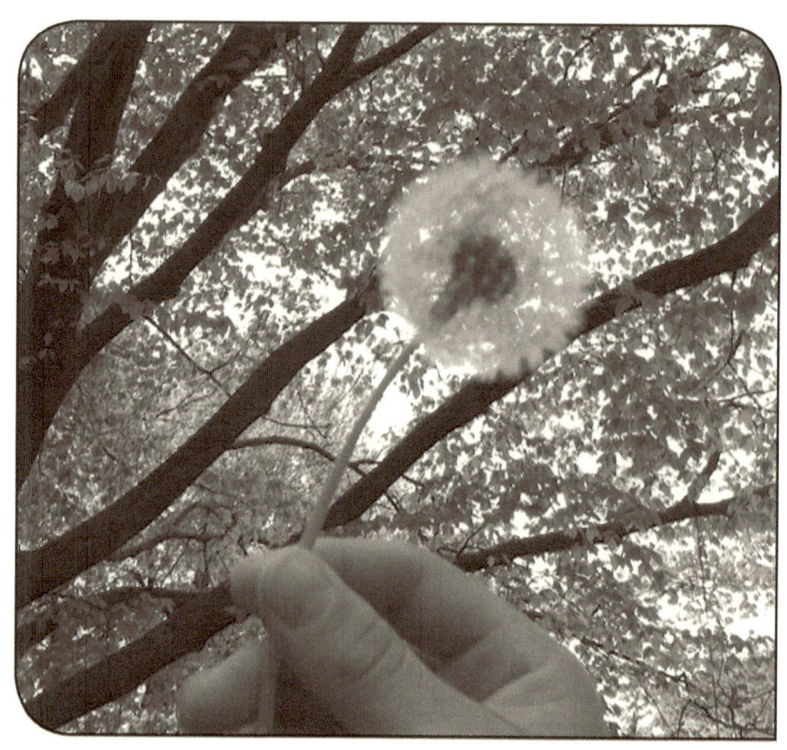

Chapter 4
Baldness Theory

What Causes Baldness/Hair Loss?

AHS causes baldness. The higher inner processing temperature of the brain, which is caused by the onset of AHS, creates the conditions for baldness. This higher nervous or internal processing frequency increases the temperature of the brain, which damages and dries the hair follicles by overheating them and depriving them of nutrients and their natural healing environment. This harsh environment damages or kills hair follicles and causes accelerated hair loss or damage.

This harsh environment can sometimes be felt as itchiness of the scalp or be visually evident in excessive sweating on the upper part of the head or in dandruff. Itchiness means that the high temperature of the brain is overheating, killing, and expelling the hair follicles. In other words, since the brain is always accelerated, it produces higher internal heat; therefore, the body no longer needs the hair for cooling. This accelerated condition causes the body to kill hair follicles and expel the hair.

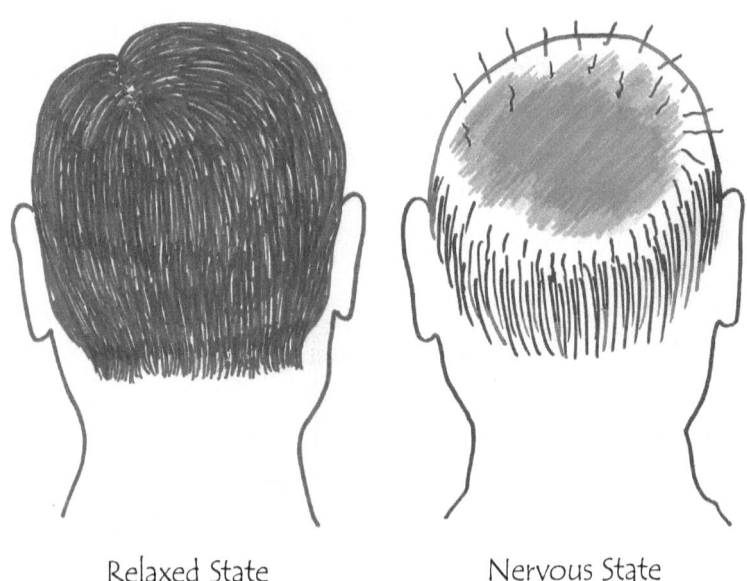

Relaxed State　　　　　　　Nervous State

Although stress can be compared to AHS it is not the same. Stress is a temporary state that comes and goes where AHS modifies the body. The meaning of the word stress has not been fully defined.

Brain-Head Hot Spots

Hair Loss

Hair loss generally starts at the crown of the head and works its way outward in a circle toward the complete upper part of the head. Once the adapted AHS process starts or stays on permanently, it generally leads to complete hair loss on the upper part of the head.

Brain Baldness Patterns

There are several baldness patterns. Baldness patterns are related to how quickly individuals adapt to AHS, how long they have AHS, their intellect, their current age, and the age when they started to adapt to AHS. For example, AHS has a greater effect on individuals with greater intellect than on others. The intellect or mental activity is determined by their environmental complexity, work demands, pace, or the type of job they are exposed to.

Complete Hair Loss from the Upper Part of the Head

This is caused when an individual has completely adapted to AHS. The body is continuously at AHS; there is no mind control or temporary reversal to the relaxed state. The brain is at a continuous nervous state, and the nerves are operating at a higher frequency and produce a higher temperature, which causes the hair follicles to dry up quickly, resulting in complete hair loss on the upper part of the head.

Hair Loss from the Frontal/Upper Part of the Head

This happens when an individual has an active and higher intellect. This is not AHS. The individual has total mind control, and the brain is not operating at a continuous nervous state. Only the hair follicles on the front of the head are affected by the controlled and heavy used of the higher processing frequency.

Hair Loss Starts at the Crown

Hair loss starts at the back upper part or crown of the head during the initial stages of adapting to AHS. The brain's nervous processing frequency begins to affect or heat up the hair follicles located around the crown area of the head. The state of mind control flips back and forth from a nervous state to a relaxed state. There are times when there is mind control, and there are times when there is no mind control over the nervous state.

Brain-Head Physical Changes

Mutations of the Head

AHS causes mutations of the head. These mutations can be seen as either the formation of a ridge on the on the upper part of the head or an overall increase in the size of the head. Unfortunately, hair loss is not the only physical change to the head resulting from AHS. The condition of over acceleration adaptation causes the brain to adapt and change. The overly active nervous system creates internal and external changes in the head. This overly active nervous condition causes the size of the brain to increase, which in turn causes the overall size of the head to increase.

This active nervous state can cause other changes to the head, including making all the hair from the rest of the head fall out because of the excessive and continuous internal nerve activity.

Hair Damage

AHS causes continuous heat; the hair follicles lose their natural healthy ambient conditions for growth. The heat hinders their purpose of cooling down the head; therefore, mutation becomes imminent and results in premature hair loss and physical change.

Detecting Changes in Hair Conditions

Changes in the hair condition can be spotted easily from the early stages of AHS to the final stages of hair loss. During the early stages, the hair reveals alternating growth sections of shiny and dry spots, which result from the mind switching between the relaxed state to a nervous state. The hair color shows alternating patterns from a dry light color to a darker healthier color every other one-sixteenth of an inch along the hair length. During the early stages of AHS, the hair recovers while an individual is sleeping or relaxing and dries up when the individual is awake and under stress. Initially, the mental state changes from a relaxed state to an AHS state, causing the hair to reveal a pattern of healthy growth and unhealthy growth. Dandruff is generally a symptom present during these early stages of AHS.

Over time, the pattern changes, causing faded or dried-up hair because of the continuous nervous state and lack of proper sleep. During the later stages of AHS, the hair becomes dull, thin, and brittle from continuous exposure to the nervous state. Faded, dull, and brittle hair requires more maintenance to keep it looking good. In comparison, healthy hair needs very little maintenance. It is flexible and bouncy and has dark solid colors; it is not affected by the use of the comb or the weather, and it is thicker.

Why Does the Hair Dry Up?

When the nervous system turns on, it produces excessive internal heat, which causes the hair to dry up. In contrast, the non-AHS condition causes the brain to produce low or normal heat, which lets the hair grow healthily. When the nervous system turns off—a condition that occurs when an individual is in a normal or relaxed state of mind—the hair recuperates. The nervous system produces internal heat—not to be confused with external heat, which is not harmful—which creates poor conditions for the hair follicles' growth and causes them to dry up from the inside.

How Does the Hair Dry Up?

This phenomenon can be seen by examining the hair carefully. The hair shows a checkerboard pattern (i.e., an on-and-off pattern coinciding with sleep and awake states) of shining light color and darker color approximately every one-sixteenth of an inch, depending on how fast the hair grows and the season of the year. The faded, dull part indicates a stressed condition, while the darker color indicates a relaxed condition. The brain initially bounces back and forth between a hyperactive state and a relaxed state, especially when an individual is sleeping, until there is a permanent onset of the hyperactive state. The permanent onset of AHS causes all the hair to become dull and faded.

Why Does the Hair Curl Up?

When the hair starts to dry up, as explained in the previous section, it becomes less flexible and less resistant to the weather, combing, or external handling. This condition of dryness of the hair causes the hair to curl up or to stay curled when combed, exposed to external conditions, or handled. Fortunately, this dryness can be remedied and the hair can recuperate when the temporary or permanent nervous condition subsides.

How to Prevent Future Hair Loss

To prevent future hair loss, an individual must complete a reversal method training course until the mind regains control of the nervous system. Reversal methods include long-term (six months or more) training to regain control of the damaging autonomic nervous energy. Once an individual regains control of the nervous energy, he or she begins to feels happy. Just by enjoying nature, he or she regains patience, loses the continuously unsatisfied appetite, and learns to speak slowly. His or her eyes do not blink continuously or they blink slowly. He or she is no longer tired, has energy, and can sleep well. The hair starts to become thick, soft, and flexible, and the scalp no longer itches. After a complete reversal, an individual feels a willingness to share his or her happiness with everyone. He or she just feels happy.

Prematurely Gray Hair

AHS causes premature aging by depriving the hair of its cool environment and by exceeding the body's ability to heal the harm that was caused from the onset of AHS or the nervous state. In other words, the higher the processing temperature of the brain, the greater the damage to the hair follicles. The heat deprives them of their nutrients and natural healing environment and therefore causes premature aging of the hair and results in gray hair.

Brain-Head Adapting to Changes

Brain Size

The size of the brain can increase, or the shape of the brain can change as a side effect of the onset of AHS and the increased nervous activity. These side effects can happen to a greater or lesser extent depending on how long AHS has been with the individual and at what age it started to become a permanent condition.

How to Permanently Recover Hair Loss

Method 1

To recover hair loss, an individual must complete a reversal method training course until the mind regains control of the nervous system. Recovery of hair loss is basically the reversal of AHS through the means of exercising to reduce the body energy and meditation to take advantage of the low energy to change the body's movements from autonomic control to mind control, especially of the smaller organ groups, such as the muscles of the eyes and those responsible for reflexive responses to external stimulation, like a loud noise. The individual needs to regain mind control and learn to slow down all muscle movements and to move only when commanded.

Method 2

Slow down the stomach energy through medication (people need to embark on research for a new medicine to help control body movements to aid this transition effort) to reduce the energy produced by the stomach without causing addiction. While under medication, the individual should take advantage of the relaxed state to change body movements from autonomic control to mind control, especially eye movements, the blinking of the eyelids, and overactive reflexes from external motivation, such as a loud noise, and to learn how to slow down and control all muscle movements at will.

These methods can get rid of the AHS and result in a recovery of healthy hair. Some hair may not return, but it can be transplanted and will survive the new relaxed and cooler scalp environment.

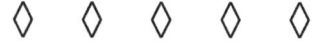

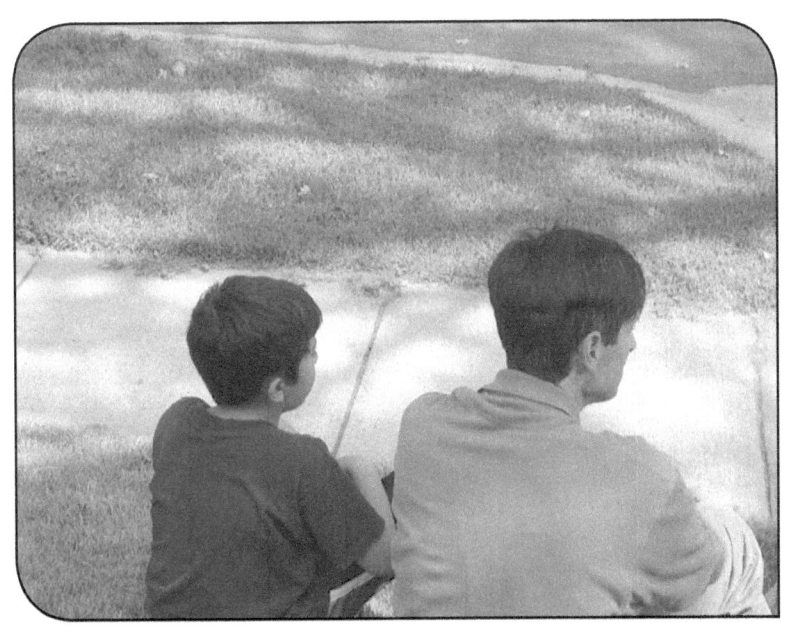

Chapter 5
Hereditary Theory

Why Does It Appear to Be Hereditary?

AHS is the onset of a nervous condition resulting from the continuous exposure to strong external stimulation of the human brain. Extensive exposure from the external media was prevalent or picked up starting in the year 1997. This condition affects young and old, men and women, and kids of all ages. Exposure to strong external media influences has continued from that time and will continue until someone makes it stop.

   The effects of the onset of this nervous condition affect individuals of different ages a little differently because of their personalities, interests, stubborn beliefs, energy levels, or just because it is more difficult to change the ways of an old man who is already set in his ways than those of a young man or a child. A young man is more likely and willing to learn and adapt to a new change since he has more energy to dispose of, he is more willing to try new ideas, he has more ambition, and he has the willingness to change the shape of his life.

The purpose of this analogy is to show that AHS has a quicker impact on the young than on the old. This analysis therefore makes it seem like the son follows the hereditary pattern of his parents, which is not true based on genes, though it is true based on exposure from living in the same household. In simple terms, the onset of a nervous condition is time sensitive, starting in the year 1997, meaning that both the child and parent are affected equally based on the start date of the external stimulation and not based on the hereditary transmission.

As an example, if we start strong external motivation on both the parent and the child at the same time, then both the parent and child will start to go bald concurrently, more or less, based on their body differences. If a parent starts to go bald at an older age, then the child will also begin to go bald at his corresponding younger age, but what actually happens is that both the parent and child are exposed to similar external stimulation from actually living in the same household or under the same roof and therefore they have similar exposure levels.

Of course, because of the conditions stated above, the child will be more likely to experience a greater effect from the external stimulation or lose his hair at a younger age because of his body constitution. In fact, however, neither the child nor the parent was meant to lose his hair at all.

Hereditary Theory

Hereditary theory promotes the idea of the transmission of learned accelerated behavior or AHS through the genes. The initial AHS state can be transmitted through the genes as an initial nervous condition only, but the effects are reversible.

Heredity and AHS
AHS can be passed through the genes—not physically but as an initial nervous state of mind only. AHS is also passed down from living in the same household and experiencing the same external exposure levels and from learning bad habits from the parent or family.

Final Stages
The final nervous state of AHS is mostly determined by the environment and not the genes. For example, if a child of an adapted AHS parent is raised in a slow environment, then he or she may reverse to the relaxed state of mind if he or she is aware of the condition.

Transmitting across Genes
Generally, the accelerated state of the parents and their environment can be passed on to the children. The child generally assumes the parents' adapted AHS or nervous state of mind.

Genes

AHS can be passed along through the genes as an initial nervous state of mind, but it is reversible or curable.

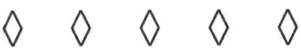

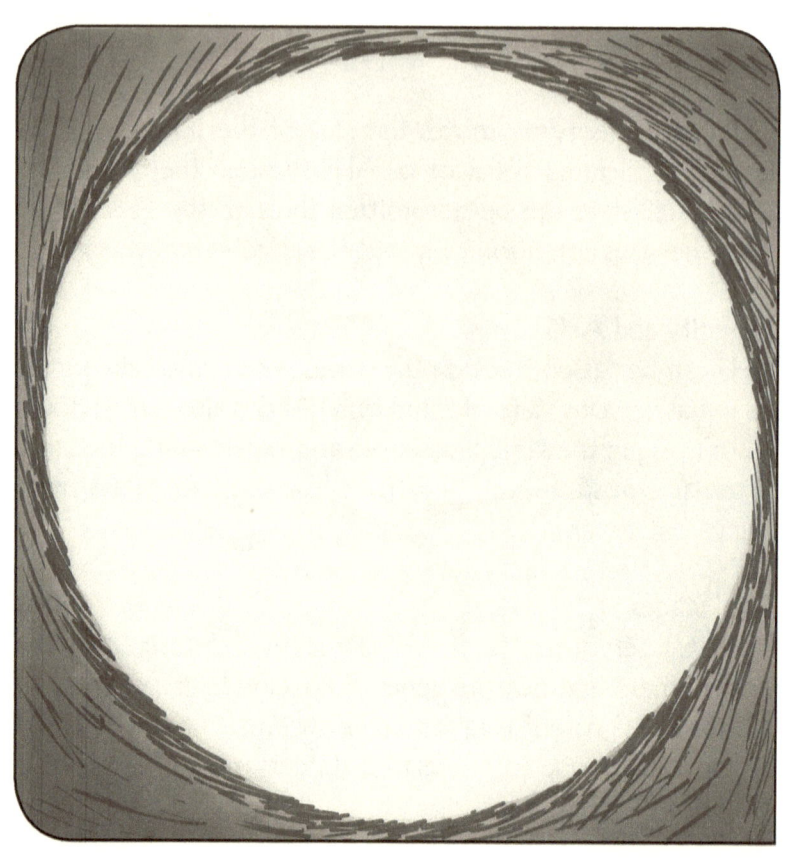

Chapter 6
Weight Gain Theory

What Makes an Individual Gain Weight?

When an individual adapts to a hyperactive condition, the body's nervous system begins to operate at a fast, uncontrollable frequency and the senses become hypersensitive. This hyperactive condition consumes and demands more energy.

The brain continuously asks for stress relief or food intake feedback more often than it normally would. The food demand is exaggerated by the hyperactive senses. The stress on the brain amplifies the needs, which must be satisfied immediately in order to avoid headaches or pain. Not only is the body using up more energy; it is also becoming more sensitive to hunger needs than normal and requires continuous and immediate satisfaction. The nerves become more sensitive or produce greater pain from hunger. To prevent this condition, an individual needs to meditate or condition the body to slow down for long periods of time to reverse to the relaxed and normal state. Then the nerves will eventually become less sensitive to hunger.

Why Do Individuals Gain Weight?

AHS is an adapted hyperactive condition that appears natural to the body, and it is practically undetectable. Once the body adapts, it stays on and consumes most of the body's inner energy. AHS uses up the body's energy faster than it can be generated; therefore, the body demands more nutrients to cope with the high-energy consumption. This high demand causes the body to stay hungry all the time.

AHS increases fatigue and stress of the mind, and, therefore, the individual requires more external gratification to relieve the stress. AHS uses up most of inner energy that the body generates, stores, and has available for exercising or playing sports. AHS stays on while an individual is sleeping, reducing his or her ability to rest, and changes his or her sleeping clock.

AHS causes the mind to stay active when it should be resting, and so an individual feels tired in the morning when he or she awakes. Since the person wakes up tired, he or she has less inner energy available during the day; he or she feels tired and loses inner energy or the drive to exercise and, as a result, gains weight. AHS also enhances the sensitivity of the nerves, which in turn exaggerates or increases the desire for food.

AHS enhances or increases the desire to consume more food, more frequently, and faster than one would without AHS or with a normal appetite. Food is needed to satisfy not only the appetite but also the exaggerated desire to eat and to relieve stress. AHS causes the stomach nerves to become overly sensitive too, and so they will produce a stronger signal to the brain, causing stress and demanding a quick response to hunger. AHS increases the sensitivity of the stomach nerves and makes the mind desperate to consume food; therefore, it is harder for an individual to control his or her appetite.

Weight Gain Based on Adapted AHS

Adapted AHS causes the body to move at an accelerated pace, so everything needs to happen fast, creating a continuous or unstoppable desire to eat or to overeat to assuage the strong appetite. Life becomes a bad habit of rushed activities associated with the continuous desire to eat, which results in overeating.

The body adapts to this nervous state or AHS condition, which causes excessive body fat and weight gain.

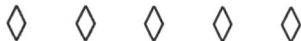

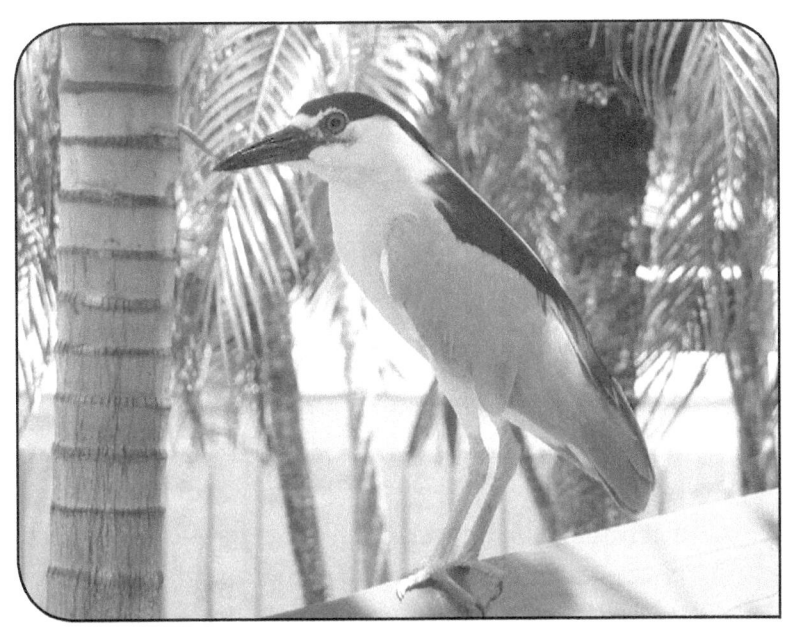

Chapter 7
Side Effects Theory

Side Effects of Chronic Hyperactive Behavior

Adaptation to AHS can cause frustration, hyperactivity, excessive aggression, oversensitivity, unhappiness, unfriendliness, strong sexual drive, and a continuous rushed state of mind.

Excessive Appetite
The high metabolism caused by AHS creates an excessive and continuously large appetite; it's almost like being continuously hungry. There is a constant urge to eat or have a tendency

to overeat. The following conditions are exaggerated by an increase in the nervous activity:

- **excessive needs/gratification**—Excessive stress requires excessive gratification.
- **hyperactivity**—Acquiring a higher body frequency causes a continuously rushed state of mind.
- **excessive sex drive**—Oversensitive nerves cause oversensitive senses and excessive sexual drive.
- **increase in allergies**—Oversensitive senses cause oversensitive allergies. The body becomes too sensitive to the environment.
- **attention deficit hyperactivity disorder**—Higher body frequency causes the loss of communication between mind control and stored memories.
- **hair dryness for women**—A higher body frequency causes excessive internal heat to be produced by the brain, which results in the hair follicles drying up and thinner hair.
- **hair loss on the top of the head for men**—A man produces a higher concentration of internal heat when compared to a woman. A higher body frequency creates excessive internal heat and causes the hair follicles to dry up and expel the hair.
- **chronic diseases**—Higher body frequency causes the loss of communication between the mind control and learned memories. The loss of communication causes the loss of body functions.

How Side Effects Materialize Differently in Different Individuals

The body constitution, genes, metabolism, strength, heart rate, and age play a major role in the ability to adapt. For example, external stimulating frequencies have a greater impact on individuals with a body frequency that closely matches the harmful external frequency. The external frequency produces more harm in individuals who can keep up or adapt to the higher external frequency.

Men versus Women

Differences in the body's constitution and nervous system play a role in the ability to adapt or mutate. Men and women have different nervous frequencies, and they release their inner energy at different rates; therefore, they respond differently to an external frequency source.

Premature Aging

Prolonged or repetitive exposure to an accelerated environment causes the body's nervous system to adapt to AHS. AHS causes premature aging. It is like keeping the car with the accelerator pedal depressed all the way down all the time—it wears out prematurely.

Premature Wrinkles

AHS causes premature wrinkles by depriving the body of the inner energy required to exercise and rejuvenate. This continuously accelerated state of mind prevents the body from accumulating the potential inner energy required to exercise and stay active. Regular body exercises are required to maintain health, stop aging, and turn the clock back in time. Regular body exercises increase the blood flow to the face and around the body and help to rebuild, recover, and rejuvenate the body's skin.

Changes in Athletes due to AHS

AHS accelerates all the body functions—breathing rate, heart rate, and so on—beyond the normal recovery or repair rate the body can provide, therefore creating an onset of body damage or wear in the form of aging and lower athletic performance or retirement at a very young age. However, AHS can enhance the performance of an overweight athlete by changing his or her performance or running speed from an expected slow running speed to an unexpected fast running speed.

Changes in Lifestyle due to AHS

Adapted AHS can reveal itself in a change of values, meaning that the onset of AHS causes the body to move at an accelerated rate, resulting in accelerated aging. Accelerated aging leads to a condition in which everything needs to happen quickly before the effects of aging set in, such as a man losing his hair, gaining weight, getting premature wrinkles or gray hair, having premature puberty, losing his looks early, getting older, and getting a sickness early; therefore, life becomes an urgency. This accelerated condition breaks the values, time line, and rules set by previous generations.

Changes in Metabolism due to AHS

As mentioned, AHS accelerates all the body's functions, including breathing rate, sweat production, inner temperature, and heart rate, beyond their normal range. The onset of hyperactivity accelerates all the body's functions, which increases the body's metabolism to the point that it damages or prematurely wears the body in the form of aging.

Changes in Energy Level due to AHS

AHS gives the body an adrenaline energy boost, which accelerates all the body functions; therefore, AHS enhances body functions and performance, which causes addition and is gratifying. Unfortunately, AHS has damaging side effects, including premature aging.

Changes in Sleep Patterns due to AHS

AHS leads to the onset of continuous nervous mental activity, which causes the mind to be active even while sleeping. Hyperactivity causes a person to sleep less at night, wake up more easily during the night, move around in bed, and wake up tired. Hyperactivity causes the mind to stay active while an individual should be sleeping; therefore, in the morning, an affected person wakes up exhausted, with irritated eyes, and stressed.

Changes in the Physical Body due to AHS

Adapted AHS can reveal itself in changes to the physical body. Meaning that the onset of AHS causes the body to mutate quicker than the normal pace, resulting in accelerated aging, loss of hair, weight gain, wrinkles, prematurely gray hair, premature puberty, and even losing the body's shape and young looks prematurely.

AHS Effects on Body Joints

AHS leads to a continuous or excessive use of the body's inner energy. This energy is expended at a faster rate than normal, which causes continuous tiredness and laziness and causes the body to become inactive for unusually long periods of time. Inactivity causes the body joints or cartilage to become weak or soft, which makes them more susceptible to damage from simple movements, such as getting up from a seated position, going down steps, or making a sudden movement.

AHS can cause excessive stress on the knee joints, which greatly reduces the amount of time an individual can stay standing up without feeling pain when compared to a relaxed person. This is caused by an oversensitive nervous system.

Loss of Patience

Adapted hyperactive condition causes the brain to be in a continuous, uncontrollable, rushed state of mind, which causes the loss of patience. Everything needs to happen fast. Since AHS cannot be slowed down, it is continuously active and running in a panic mode all the time; the lack of activity causes stress, and patience is lost.

AHS Effect on Age Group

Age group effects how quickly the onset of AHS can

occur in an individual based on the body's energy level and constitution. The initial state of mind, energy level, activity level, mind control, learned behaviors, and other factors affect how quickly an individual can adapt and how fast the onset of AHS can occur.

Detecting Changes

Changes can manifest in the following conditions: the hair beginning to dry up, a strong and frequently elevated appetite, a short temper, a lack of patience, a loss of admiration for nature, time passing by too fast, allergies, overly sensitive nerves, weight gain, premature aging, loss of concentration, fast talking, rushed attitude, excessive blinking of the eyes, unsteady hands, shaking of the hand when the arm is extended, excessive perspiration, feeling hot all the time, a continuous desire for gratification, sudden movements, panic attacks, stressed condition, premature puberty, excessive child growth, a "me only" attitude, hatred toward society, lack of mental concentration, lack of creativity, inability to stand up for long periods of time, pain in the knees, and jerky body movements, like digital signals or on/off signals versus gradual movements.

Changes over a One-Year Period

Side Effects

Typical side effects from the start of AHS over a one-year period consist of hair dryness, itchy scalp, dandruff, increase in hair loss, and a loss of body control; an individual tends to bump into things and make mistakes while talking. He or she also experiences an increase in appetite, a lack of sleep, a fast laugh, weight gain, and a continuous hyperactive or rushed state.

Face Skin Tone Changes

The skin pattern of some individuals with AHS has an unnaturally fluffy baby-like skin tone on the face with excessive fat from the increased food consumption, blood flow, and nerve activity in the face. These fluffier skin conditions can also surface on other parts of the body, depending on how the nervous condition manifests itself in an individual.

Long-Term Effects and Aging

Physical Changes

Adapted AHS can reveal itself in permanent physical changes, meaning that the onset of AHS causes the body to mutate at an accelerated pace, resulting in long-term side effects. The face changes—concave cheeks become fat cheeks. The head changes from having a full head of hair to complete hair loss on the top of the head. The body changes from a trim fit to a full look; body joints decay prematurely, the size of the head increases, women get wrinkles prematurely, and people get gray hair or undergo premature puberty. People lose their looks early. Dark circles appear around the eyes, and people get chronic diseases.

AHS accelerates all the body's functions beyond the normal recovery or repair rate that the body can provide, creating the onset of body damage or wear in the form of aging.

Increased Tension

AHS causes an uncontrollable, accelerated pace. Patience is lost, and an individual can no longer slow down. Everything needs to happen more quickly. The biological clock has been accelerated, and anything other than superfast speed causes mental tension and results in the loss of mental control.

Positive/Negative Effects on Learned Behavior

AHS may have some positive effects. It can help a mentally slow child to become more mentally active, which may help an individual to live independently and meet the demands of our fast-paced and demanding society.

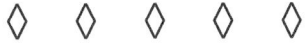

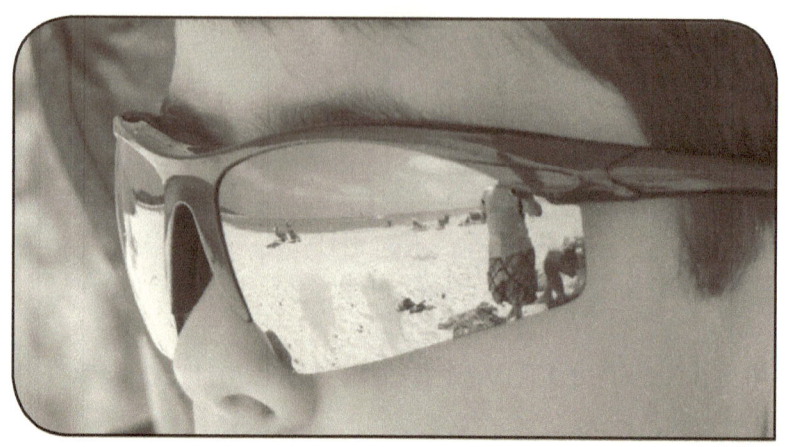

Chapter 8
Environment Theory

Environment and AHS

Environmental Impact
The fast-moving environment can cause AHS. The quick flipping of commercials shown on TV can turn on the nervous system and result in a permanent or continuous onset of a nervous state of mind. The eyes and mind try to keep up with the speed of the commercials, which are faster than the natural frequency of the human brain. These fast-moving commercials cause the mind to turn on the faster nervous frequency in order to keep up and be able to see the rapidly flipping scenes. Minimize watching commercials when the screens are flipping very fast.

Defining the Environment
Environment is the external influence that affects or turns on

the nervous trigger. Fast-moving TV commercials, computer games, and other electronic devices can trigger the autonomic inner nervous energy to keep up with the speed demand. Prolonged use of this nervous energy causes the onset of the AHS condition.

TV and the Environment

The quick flipping of commercials shown on TV or fast-moving computer games can unconsciously turn on the autonomic nervous system. This happens because the eyes and mind try to keep up with the flickering speed of commercials on TV, which are faster than the natural frequency of the human brain. Continuous exposure to this type of external motivation can cause the onset of AHS.

Minimize watching commercials when the screens are flickering very fast. The speed of commercials has substantially increased over the years. To validate this observation, compare commercials that were created pre-1997 with commercials that were created post-1997.

Environment-Induced Motivation

External influence can unconsciously turn on the autonomic system or nervous mechanism of the brain. Prolonged and repetitive exposure to accelerated external motivation plays an important role in how quickly AHS sets in.

Self-Induced Motivation

Self-induced motivation is the process that causes an individual to consciously trigger or turn on the autonomic or nervous mechanism of the brain in order to extend the abilities or perform better. Conscious motivation, such as stimulants and other medical accelerators, play an important role in how quickly AHS sets in.

Environment Directly Related to AHS

External accelerated or rushed influence can trigger the body's autonomic mechanism or nervous trigger. Repetitive exposure to an external accelerated or rushed work environment causes this repetitive use of the nervous trigger, which eventually stays on permanently.

The Laws of Equality across Ages

The Laws of Equality
AHS is mostly caused by influences from the environment that affect the young, old, and individuals from different genders and ethnic groups. The effects differ depending on the body's ability to learn and adapt to an external influence; therefore, the effects may appear to differ, but they all lead sooner or later to the same outcome—AHS.

The external influence consists of high-frequency external media and games, fast-paced work environments, influences from already affected coworkers and friends, and a high-stress external environment. All these factors contribute to how fast an individual acquires AHS and how well an individual can deal with AHS. For some individuals, it may seem like a new normal AHS state, while for others, it can be manifested as a devastating physical (sickness, weight gain) or psychological (panic, unstable) condition.

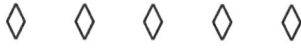

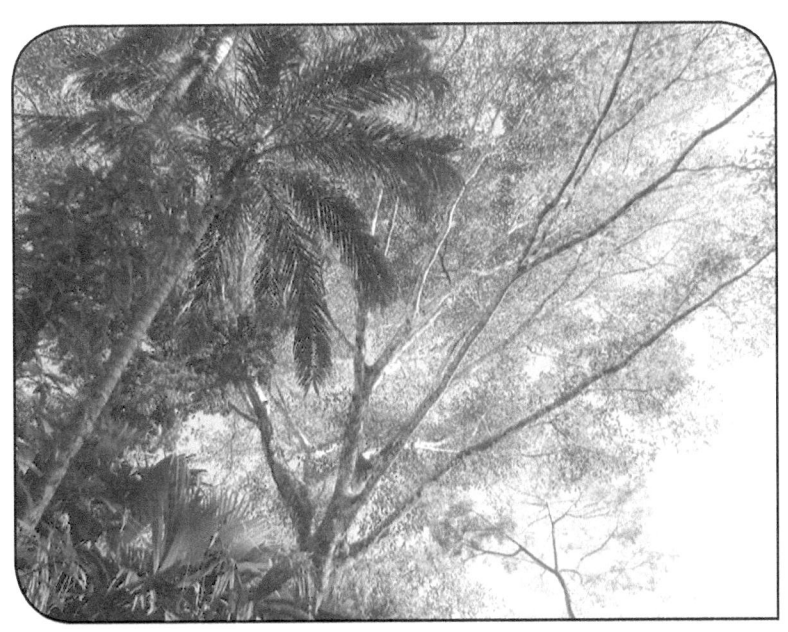

Chapter 9
Chronic Conditions, Diseases, and the Immune System

Effects of Sickness on the Immune System

When the body is sick or is fighting an infection, the immune system is overtaxed and therefore is too weak to fight other infections concurrently. Do not let any type of sickness stay in the body for more than two weeks. After two weeks, the body starts to adapt or change to support the disease.

Exercise to get rid of a sickness and to strengthen the immune system; relax, eat well, and take the correct antibiotics at the proper time during the day. Help support the benefits of antibiotics by eliminating stress and alcohol during the sick period.

Help Medicine Help the Disease

Help medicine help the disease. While taking antibiotics for an infection, try to stay calm and in a stress-free environment; stay away from external media even when you are beginning to feel better. Relaxation helps the medicine have a greater success rate, especially when an individual has a very weak immune system. Regain control of the mind by walking, going outdoors, painting, or employing a slow, constructive mental activity.

While taking relaxing medicines for migraines, try to stay active in a slow-paced, stress-free, or relaxed state, even though taking the medicine may generate lots of inner energy for the body to spend. This relaxation process helps the medicine do its job to get rid of the pain and prevent future illness.

The Stomach Supports the Immune System

The effectiveness of the immune system begins with how the stomach processes food. Keep the stomach healthy so that the immune system stays healthy. Exercise, eat healthy food, and relax in order to keep the stomach healthy. Take apple vinegar to kill a stomach virus.

Brain Processing Frequency-Communication with the Body—Disorders

Learning Disabilities
The onset of a disability is dependent on when or at what point

in his or her lifetime an individual adapts to AHS or if the mind has enough time to learn this new condition. The onset is also dependent on the individual's ability to find and retrieve old learned memories. Lifelong memories are stored in the brain at the slower normal frequency and are needed to perform basic body movements and functions. The quick onset of AHS can lead to attention deficit hyperactivity disorder and Parkinson's and Alzheimer's diseases. The quick onset of AHS causes the mind to lose access rapidly to memories that were stored at the original natural frequency and are needed to control and operate body functions.

Parkinson's Disease

The individual loses the ability to access the natural frequency of the brain needed to perform basic body movements. This is probably due to the loss of communication between the body and the brain when the communicating frequency increases above the normal frequency. The higher frequency becomes the norm and can no longer access memories that were stored at the lower frequency, including learned behaviors, such as walking and other functions. This can basically be referred to as an adapted attention deficit hyperactivity disorder at an old age.

Alzheimer's Disease

Alzheimer's is similar to Parkinson's except the loss in communication affects primarily the memory frequency. This is similar to Parkinson's where the loss of communication is an extension of using the wrong frequency to retrieve saved memories. This can also be referred to as attention deficit hyperactivity disorder of an old age. An older individual cannot adapt as easily as a younger individual to this change in state, especially if the transition happens quickly and the condition is not understood.

Attention Deficit Hyperactivity Disorder (ADHD)

ADHD is the loss of the body's ability to retrieve old memories at a young age. The body loses its ability to retrieve old memories when it changes, and memories that were saved in the brain at a lower frequency are being retrieved at a different or a higher frequency. This is similar to Parkinson's where the body's frequency changes or the communication frequency changes, which decreases the body's ability to retrieve the saved memories. A young individual, unlike an older individual, can adapt and recreate new connections and make new memories in the brain to allow the mind to learn and regain control of the body's functions and to make use of new memories.

Stress and Migraines

Stress is a temporary forced link or connection between the mind's control and the autonomic or nervous system in its accelerated or hyperactive state for a short period of time.

In a hyperactive individual, the mind is generally either not connected or connected for short periods of time to the accelerated nervous system. Stress occurs when the mind is forced to gain control of an adapted hyperactive state or accelerated nervous system for a longer period of time than typical. This causes the mind to accelerate to keep up with the nervous system, which generates stress. In a relaxed individual, stress is caused when the mind control, which is normally connected to the nervous system, is forced to stay temporarily connected while the nervous system is temporarily accelerated, such as during a meeting or a presentation.

Stress is a temporary connection between two dissimilar processing frequencies: mind control and the accelerated or hyperactive state of the nervous system. The mind control is being forced to accelerate in order to process and analyze an enormous amount of data and several commands at the higher frequency of the autonomic nervous system. The mind control is temporarily connected to a hyperactive nervous state. Stress generally subsides when the link is broken or the nervous system slows down.

These types of connections could lead to migraines, nausea, loose stomach, and stress. Currently, the permanent onset of AHS is not considered stress since the body adapts to this condition, and since it feels natural, it cannot be easily diagnosed. In this book, the word *stress* is defined to differentiate from the recovery theory, which is the permanent onset of a hyperactive state or AHS.

What causes a migraine? The answer is the lack of oxygen to the brain. The above hyperactive conditions cause the brain and body to be out of balance. This means that under a hyperactive condition, the brain requires a greater supply of oxygen from the blood. If the individual is not breathing enough oxygen and the blood has a low percentage of oxygen or if the veins shrink and there is a reduced flow of blood, the brain is deprived of oxygen and this can cause a migraine. How can an individual prevent a migraine? The answer is to be aware when one is in a stressful condition and start breathing exercises through the nose. The migraine symptoms will go away half an hour after the exercises. There are many conditions that can reduce the delivery of oxygen to the brain, for example, exercise, humidity, altitude, pressure, heart conditions, hormone imbalances, etc.

Is Stress a Disease?

Although stress can be compared to AHS it is not the same. Stress is a temporary state that comes and goes where AHS modifies the body. If Parkinson's, Alzheimer's, obesity, and attention deficit hyperactivity disorder are diseases, then the permanent onset of hyperactivity or adapted AHS is also a disease. The temporary onset of stress is not a disease. Stress is not a disease until it becomes a chronic or permanent condition. AHS is a chronic or permanent hyperactive state of the mind and body.

Effects of Stress on the Immune System

The effectiveness of the immune system begins with how the stomach processes food. Stress excites the nerves going to the stomach, which can weaken or hinder the stomach's ability to process food needed to create immune system. Adapted AHS or turning on the autonomic nervous mechanism causes continuous strain on the stomach, which can reduce or prevent the stomach's ability to the process food needed to create the immune system necessary to protect the body from diseases.

What Is a Chronic Condition?

A chronic condition is the permanent onset of an accelerated hyperactive state of mind, which is caused when the nervous system is continuously turned on and the organs adapt. It is linked to all the body functions. This is an adapted state of mind, which was caused by the repetitive use of the nervous trigger in response to a vigorous or emergency condition.

This adapted state causes a fast-paced way of life that cannot be slowed down or turned off.

Chronic behavior is basically a learned or AHS condition. This adapted condition can result in lifelong conditions, which are referred to as diseases. These chronic conditions are reversible.

AHS Effects on Alzheimer's and Parkinson's

Chronic conditions are reversible. The older an individual is and the longer he or she has had the condition, the harder it will be to reverse, since there may be some permanent damage to the brain from the abuse caused by the adapted AHS condition.

AHS Effects on Heart Attacks

AHS could lead to decreased physical activity, overeating, stress, and continuous fatigue. These are conditions that can lead to heart attacks. Along with the above attributes, heart attacks can occur when the mind locks into and stays in a harmful resonance frequency, stuck between the relaxed frequency and the hyperactive frequency of the body. This resonance frequency causes excessive stress and requires a high blood demand; at the same time, it does not allow the body to process food properly. This harmful condition occurs when the body changes in frequency from a relaxed frequency to a hyperactive one or from a hyperactive frequency to a relaxed one. Increasing or decreasing the body frequency above or below the resonance frequency can prevent a heart attack by reducing mental stress and increasing the blood supply to the brain. High-stress conditions generally occur late at night while sleeping or early in the morning while waking up when mental stress is at the highest. Medications with caffeine and aspirin, such as Excedrin, can reduce stress by reducing the blood viscosity and therefore increasing the blood flow to the brain. Also mild body torso flexing exercises (five hundred) can decrease mental frequency.

AHS Effects on the Immune System

An AHS-adapted nervous condition could weaken the immune system. Adapted AHS weakens the stomach and its ability to produce antibodies or the immune system. It can also cause it to overproduce antibodies, which can result in a harmful or an overactive immune system.

AHS Effects on Child Growth

In the same way that AHS enhances (or accelerates) the body functions, it also accelerates, enhances, or overstimulates the sensors, which regulate the body's natural growth mechanism. These oversensitive nerves increase the body's growth process the same way that the organs of a man can grow after maturity.

Childhood Hyperactivity or Attention Deficit Hyperactivity Disorder

Attention deficit hyperactivity disorder is a loss of the body's ability to retrieve memories, which were stored at the lower normal frequency rate prior to the onset of AHS. AHS operates at a higher frequency, which is not compatible with the lower normal frequency at which the memories were initially stored; this incompatibility causes intermittent memory lapses.

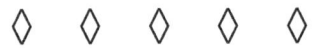

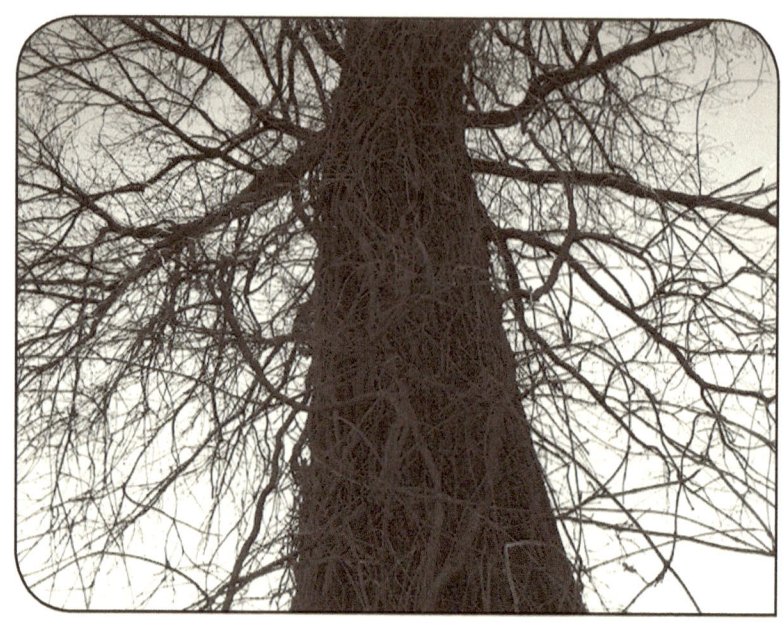

Chapter 10
Adaptation Theory

How Changes Occur

Main Causes

Adaptation can occur from repetitive exposure to a harmful environment, such as working in a fast-paced job or living under fear or threat. The body uses its inner nervous energy in order to keep up with the high demand or accelerated pace or to protect itself from harm. The nervous system adapts to survive.

Remedies
Removing the harmful environment assists with the reversal process.

Time Line
Adaptation to AHS can occur in as little as six months to one year. Reversal can take as long as one to three years, depending on external influences or the environment. I am hopeful that a new type of medication, along with new relaxing techniques, can lead to a quicker reversal time line.

Typical Sequence to AHS

Start
Adaptation can start from the influence of the external environment or self-motivation.

Two Weeks
Adaptation starts revealing itself in a flip-flop mode in which the mind goes in and out of the stressed state. During this stressed or nervous state, the hair begins to dry up. The hair shows sequential sections of dried-up shiny rings and sections of darker, healthy hair. The hair rejuvenates while one is sleeping or during the slow periods and creates a healthy darker ring. The hair dries up while one is awake or during the accelerated periods and creates a dried-up shiny ring.

Hair grows healthily while an individual has a good night's sleep. The inner temperature of the brain stays cool, nourishing the hair and creating a healthy ring or section of the hair. During the day, when the brain is accelerated, it produces excessive heat to the hair follicle, creating a nonnourishing, hot, and unhealthy environment, which causes dried-up rings to form in those sections of the hair that grew under these harsh conditions.

During the nervous state of mind, the hair grows and develops shiny, dried-up rings, while during the relaxed state of mind, the hair grows and develops darker healthy rings. Corresponding to periods of nervous and relaxed states of the mind, the hair shows a pattern of dried and healthy rings along its length. During the nervous state, the brain generates excessive heat from the continuous nervous activity. The hot inner temperature of the brain heats up and kills the hair follicle and expels the hair.

One Month
Adaptation reveals itself in uncontrollable behavior, lack of sleep, and more dryness in the hair, though there are still some healthy ring sections.

Six Months
Adaptation reveals itself in the solid, shiny dryness of the hair and some hair loss, circles under the eyes, lack of sleep, continuous tiredness, impatience, and a rushed state.

One Year
Adaptation reveals itself as dryness of the hair with more hair loss, circles under the eyes, lack of sleep, continuous tiredness, impatience, a rushed state, frustration, and unhappiness.

Three Years
Adaptation reveals itself as excessive hair loss, weight gain, allergic reactions, loss of feelings and emotions, fatigue, lack of energy, impatience, rushing, frustration, and unhappiness. The mind and body learn to cope with the new rushed state of mind.

Changes in the Metabolism due to Adapted AHS

Changes in the metabolism can be detected by a sudden increase in one's appetite and eating frequency between meals, impatience, lack of sleep, loss of patience, dandruff, itchiness on the scalp, hair loss, premature aging, premature gray hair, excessive weight gain, rapid eye movement, loss of concentration, nervous energy, inability to relax, frustration, hyperactivity, aggression, oversensitivity, and excessive sexual drive.

Human Mutation Theory

The body and mind can unconsciously memorize a particular nervous state when the mind is exposed for long enough. The mind can memorize a stressful condition, a disease, a fast way of talking, a harsh environment, a fast-paced environment, an unpleasant environment, a rude environment, or a hostile environment to the point that the body changes to adapt to the new environment.

The body and mind change to adapt to new conditions; if exposed for long periods of time, they can stay permanently in that nervous state of mind. This new adapted state of mind can lead to premature mutation of the body. Over time, the body is physically altered, the head gets bigger, and an individual tends to gain weight and lose hair. The metabolism changes, and the body changes physically or mutates from the predicted normal or hereditary condition.

Long-Term Consequences

Long-term side effects can be seen as excessive weight gain, loss of patience, baldness, premature aging, premature gray hair, an unfriendly attitude, nervous energy, an inability to relax, lack of sleep, circles around the eyes, frustration, hyperactivity, over aggression, oversensitivity, a loose stomach, and allergies.

Consequences over Time

Side effects or changes to the body can result from an adapted AHS condition. AHS initially appears gratifying or satisfying because of the excessive adrenaline or rush of energy through the body. The mind and body learn to speed up because it is gratifying, but over time, unforeseen harmful or undesirable side effects, such as premature aging, hair loss, and weight gain, reveal themselves.

Short-Term Effects of Relaxation

Relaxation cannot be accomplished over short periods of time. Most relaxation techniques, such as yoga, are currently employed for short periods, and therefore they are ineffective in controlling the long-term onset of AHS. Please note that AHS is a chronic condition and requires long-term meditation and controlled relaxation techniques to reverse it.

The controlled relaxation period needs to match the stress period, probably up to six months or more, to allow the body to adapt and learn the new nervous state of mind. The time frame to adapt to a relaxed state changes depending on the body's ability to control the autonomic nervous system.

Relaxation occurs when the mind finally takes control of the autonomic nervous system.

Accelerated Mutation and AHS

Accelerated Mutation

AHS accelerates mutation of the body. The body can start to mutate in as little as one year. The body adapts to survive, even in a harsh environment, when exposed for a prolonged period of time. The same way that AHS enhances (or accelerates) body functions, it can also accelerate, enhance, or overstimulate the body's senses, which regulate the body's natural growth mechanism. This AHS condition breaks down our basic understanding of mutation and alters our existing laws of nature on evolution.

Mutation

AHS can lead to premature body mutation in as little time as six months to a year.

Getting Older and Gaining Stress

When individuals get older, he or she exercises and goes out less, which causes him or her to keep the stress from work inside rather than to release it. This regular unhealthy conditioning of the body results in a gradual increase in stress that can lead to adapted AHS. This adaptation condition makes older individuals very susceptible to chronic or nervous diseases at an old age.

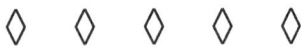

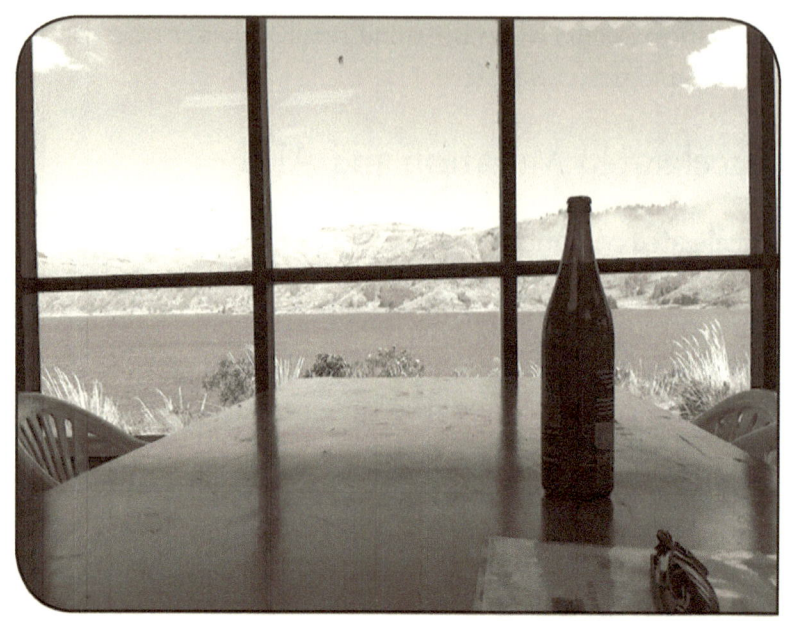

Chapter 11
Analysis Theory

Research Technique

Additional studies may be necessary to discover other techniques or medicines to aid or reduce the recovery process time line. To prove the theory, a research protocol can be designed as a year-plus-long study with a group of twenty to thirty individuals (male subjects ages ten to forty years old) in a low-frequency or artificially controlled environment.

Many factors can be monitored, including the initial state of health. Document the following individual activities at the beginning and during the study;

likes and dislikes;
daily activity level;
daily exercises;
number of hours per day spent playing computer or portable device games, texting, surfing the Internet, or watching television;
food intake;
type of food;
perspiration level;
sleeping patterns;
eye movements;
sexual attraction;
pornography inclinations;
goals;
health status,
heart condition,
cholesterol level,
panic conditions;
type of sports played;
competitive level of sports;
and so on;

Document the body conditions at the beginning and during of the study;

body size;
magnified pictures of their natural or untreated hair color from selected parts of the head;
hair history by interview or through pictures at different ages since birth; immediate family hair history;
body energy level;
age group;

allergies;
skin problems;
male/female

Document the data at home, work and household at the beginning and during the study;

type of work;
entertainment;
hobbies;
reading habits
household members;
parents' behavior patterns;
Simple tools may be used to measure all the dimensions of each individual to define the realms of his or her life.

The result of each dimension can be organized into numerous files, and the result may be measurements of changes based on hair conditions, including fields based on hair templates designed for each individual and entered and interpreted by a trained observer over the specified period.

The study should include a mechanical equipment test conducted before and after the year-long conditioning therapy (e.g., a test for patience by assembling a lengthy, delicate, and complicated mechanical system to measure patience, precision, accuracy, and mind control).

What Happens after a Complete Reversal?

Reversal methods result over a long-term period, six months or more (it took me three years to achieve a complete reversal), of training the body to regain control or slow down the damaging autonomic energy until the natural feeling of happiness returns, there is an appreciation for nature, patience is renewed, the continuous appetite subsides, the person learns to speak slowly, and the eyes naturally do not blink or blink slowly. The individual is no longer tired, has energy, and sleeps well. The hair is soft and flexible, the scalp no longer itches, and there is a desire to share the happiness with everyone. He or she just feels happy. Please note that a quick reversal is not recommended, since it may lead to health problems. The body organs will need to be conditioned to support the new relaxed condition, including processing of cholesterol.

Working without AHS

The mind can be more productive in a working environment without AHS. It is more creative and intelligent and therefore produces more accurate and better results. To achieve a higher level of productivity, an individual must work at a frequency just shy of the body's AHS frequency. An individual can be faster and more productive by eliminating compulsive or automatic actions that may require reworking. Staying just shy of the AHS frequency allows the mind to control and process accurate information and at the same time maintain control of the autonomic nervous system.

The turning on of the nervous system takes place when the body's actions match the nervous frequency. It creates strong pulsating digital signals along with a rush of adrenaline that stays on even when an individual has long tried to stop the nervous activity. The nervous system can easily be turned on, but it is very difficult to turn off.

Knowing the Difference between AHS and Not AHS

AHS changes the nervous system. It causes hypersensitivity. There is less mental control and more autonomic control. More gratification is needed to satisfy sensitive nerves. The nerves are more sensitive to pain and the environment, and since the nerves are more sensitive, allergies are more common. Non-AHS is the condition when an individual feels happy just enjoying nature; he or she has patience, does not have a continuous appetite, and speaks and laughs slowly. His or her eyelids do not blink unconsciously or blink slowly. He or she is no longer tired in the morning and has continuous inner energy. The hair stays soft and flexible. The scalp no longer itches. He or she feels a willingness to share his or her happiness with everyone. He or she just feels happy.

How to Stay Away from AHS

AHS is caused by a fast-paced environment. Unfortunately, it is man-made. Stay away from the man-made environment or external rushed or accelerated influences. Go outdoors to the wilderness, exercise, make or create things with the hands, help others, slow down, change the attitude from "for me" to "for others," and stay happy.

How to Determine If an Individual Has AHS

Changes in the metabolism can be detected by an increase in appetite, increased frequency of snacking between meals, impatience, lack of sleep, dandruff, itchiness on the scalp, premature hair loss, excessive hair loss, premature aging, premature gray hair, excessive weight gain, rapid eye movement, continuous eye burning and blinking, lack of concentration, nervous energy, increase in body temperature, feeling hot, excessive sweating, tiredness, inability to relax, frustration, hyperactivity, excessive aggression, oversensitivity, rushed state of mind, need for alcohol, need for stress medication, uncontrollable children, a continuous need for material gratification, excessive sexual activity, allergies, and a be-the-first or look-out-for-number-one attitude.

The nervous system can impair the five body senses by increasing the nerve sensitivity and feedback signal strength, which exaggerates the body's needs or demands going to the mind.

How an Individual Feels If He or She Does Not Have AHS?

A mind at peace means a state of mind in which happiness occurs constantly without the need for material things or food for long periods of time. It is a state where boredom is not frustrating. There is a state of patience, gentleness, helpfulness, gratitude, sensitivity, wanting to share the joy, and friendliness. An individual gains control of his or her emotions and feelings, such as sexual desire and hunger, and has an increase in the tolerance for pain. The nerves associated with the five senses are under the mind's control; therefore, the senses associated with hunger, sex, and feelings are reduced.

Men versus Women Theory

The man's body design allows the release of his inner energy quickly over a short period of time, while the woman's body design allows the release of the inner energy slowly over a longer time period. This difference (hormones) causes the man to induce greater heat and damage to the hair follicles during AHS, and therefore the man is prone to premature hair loss.

Men and women are different; women have quicker reflexes and a higher mental frequency, which therefore can cope better and more naturally with fast-paced external demands or motivation without having to tap into the inner nervous energy; therefore, they have the ability to stay calm under a high-pressure demand. Men have an enormous amount of energy that they can release in a very short time, giving them a lot of power, but it has less long-term endurance.

Why does this matter? Men's explosive power and quick release of energy when under AHS cause excessive heat in the upper part of the brain, resulting in quick hair loss. Women, on the other hand, slowly release energy, even under AHS. This generates less heat, which causes less damage to the hair follicles. Also keep in mind that not all men and women have the same constitution. Some men have less of the male hormones, which causes them to have more moderate reactions, and some women have more aggressive reactions.

Men and women adapt to a fast external environment in different ways. Adaptation for a man reveals itself as excessive hair loss and weight gain, while adaptation for a woman may reveal itself as weight gain, premature aging, and excessive dryness of the hair.

Classification of AHS Based on Age Group

When in the life span of an individual the onset of AHS

occurred plays a critical role in developing a reversal plan. Individuals who developed AHS at an earlier stage in their lives will require a reversal plan structure with more rigorous exercises and meditation techniques for a longer reversal period than individuals in whom the onset occurred later in life or at an older age.

For an eighteen-year-old male who started to lose some hair during the last year, has dried-up hair or dandruff and an itchy scalp, or has curly hair on the crown and forehead, see the guidelines in the next chapter to quickly stop hair loss and to start gaining new hair.

Other groups are classified as follows:

⬧ male, twelve to eighteen years
⬧ male, twelve and under
⬧ male, nineteen to forty
⬧ male forty-one to sixty-five
⬧ the same age groups for women and for groups based on country of origin

The length of the reversal period will change depending on which classification group an individual belongs to.

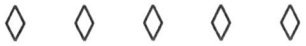

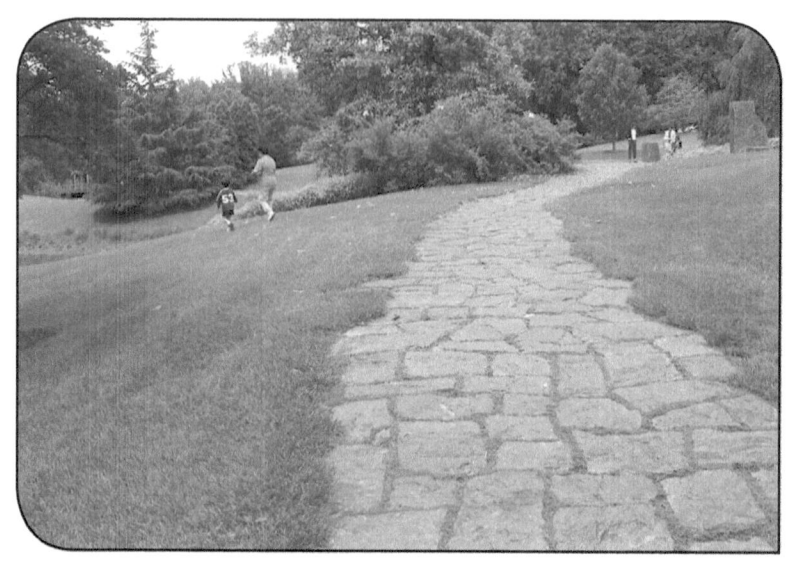

Chapter 12
Reversal Theory

Reversal Theory Time Line

AHS can be reversed through continuous controlled meditation efforts over a period of one to three years without external accelerated influence. This reversal period might be reduced to six months with medication, depending on the condition or mental state of the individual. The reversal process will not happen by itself or by cutting off harmful external motivation, since the body has already learned this new AHS condition. There has to be a self-motivated willingness to try to slow the body down in order to change back from a hyperactive state to a relaxed state. Please note that a quick reversal is not recommended, since it may lead to health problems. The body organs will need to be conditioned to support the new relaxed condition, including the processing of cholesterol.

Reversal Methods

Green Guidelines

Reversal refers to the process of training the body back to the unstressed condition by regaining control of the autonomic energy. Use the following basic methods throughout the day:

1. Start to practice controlling blinking your eyes and restricting your eyelids to move only when commanded; even if your eyes are burning, only blink on command and then blink slowly; try to do this throughout the day and even at night while sleeping. Excessive blinking of the eyelids creates dark circles under the eyes.

2. Learn to control the panic energy by not responding to loud noises. Do not move when you hear a loud sound; first, analyze the noise, and move only after the signal has been analyzed and the body has been Practice moving the arms and fingers only after they have been commanded to move.

3. Reversal methods require practicing the methods listed above throughout the day for the long term, six months or more, training to regain control of the damaging autonomic nervous energy. Exercise, if possible, prior to performing the techniques listed above to reduce the inner energy of the body and allow for easier mind control.

Other Important Green Guidelines

1. Become fully aware of your body movements consistently throughout the day.
2. Move only after the signal has been analyzed and the body has been commanded to move.
3. Do not watch fast-moving external media.
4. Stay away from pornographic media and events.
5. Perform extensive exercise for long periods of time (two hours per day) more or less, depending on the individual's physical condition. Exercise is one of the only ways to calm down the nervous system. Stay relaxed while exercising by trying to think slow, pleasant thoughts. An individual can move as fast as he wants during the exercise, but it is important to maintain a slow mind.
6. Do not go to sleep when the eyes are burning or they feel tired. In reality, the body is not tired, but the burning of the eyes clouds the judgment and makes the mind believe that the body is actually exhausted. Generally, this type of tiredness is caused by stress and prevents an individual from getting a good night's sleep. Meditate or perform light or slow exercises before going to sleep. Perform exercises, such as light torso movement and going out to walk around the neighborhood. It is better to sleep later with exercise than to sleep earlier, under stress, without exercise.
7. Do not look at everything or everyone you see, even while driving. Slow down the movements of the eyes. Move naturally like an analog system rather than like a digital system. An analog system moves gradually

from a low to a greater signal while digital signals are instantaneous; they change from on to off instantly.

8. Move the eyes slowly to change from one view to another.

9. Move the eyes slowly while reading. Move the eyes slowly when changing from one word to another word.

10. Minimize worrying about unnecessary things.

11. Do not overreact to loud noises or alarms. Move only after the situation has been analyzed and action is required.

12. Try staring at an object for a long period of time without blinking. This process allows the mind to learn to control nervous eye movements. Practice regularly to increase or gain control.

13. Minimize the use of medications and alcohol, unless necessary. It is very difficult to control the body when the mind is being altered by medication.

14. Condition the body to learn, function, operate, and stay at a slow frequency.

15. Try to stay in places where things are moving slowly.

16. Try speaking slowly by not rushing the words. It can be proven that speaking quickly is caused by an overdose of stress from a fast work environment and overexposure to fast media devices.

17. Try thinking slowly by minimizing the number of thoughts in the head. Try focusing on slow thoughts (floating on water, painting the walls, taking long walks, etc.).

18. Watch old-fashioned, or some even recent, slow movies, such as *The Natural* and *Les Miserables*.

Perform these green guidelines from six months up to

three years until the mind feels happy when just enjoying nature, patience is regained, there is no longer a continuous appetite, the mind has been conditioned to speaking slowly, the eyes naturally do not blink or blink slowly, the mind is no longer tired and the body has energy, sleeping is good, the hair is soft and flexible, the scalp no longer itches, and there is a desire to share the happiness with everyone. Exercising is the best way to stabilize the body's energy level and make it easier to control the inner energy with meditation along with slow movement techniques until reversal adaptation takes place.

Reversing the Human Mutation Theory

Reversing AHS is the process to regain control of the body's autonomic nervous system. A permanent change to the nervous system can be reversed through controlled long-term meditation and slow mind control exercises. The mind needs to regain control of the autonomic nervous system. The mind and body need to be removed from a rushed or accelerated external environment until control is regained.

How Long to Reverse Adaptation?

Reversing an adapted system can take as long as six months, one year, or three years under meditated mind control, depending on the person's ability to learn and adapt, if he or she is removed from a rushed or accelerated external environment. The mind learns by doing.

Reversing an adapted system needs to be done with the correct meditation techniques. The final goal is to achieve control of the autonomic nervous system so that it can be slowed down. The goal is to have every part of the body move only when commanded. There should be no nervous or uncontrolled movement. Try not to take any medicines, such as stimulants, that accelerate the nervous system. Try practicing the following seven meditation techniques and use them throughout the day.

1. Work on staring at one object without blinking, moving the eyelids, moving the eyes, or changing the focus, and do this without thinking about anything. The eyes will tend to blink, burn, or try to change focus. Perform eye-control exercises for half an hour or more per day until eye movement control is regained. You will not be able to achieve this eyes control state until you are totally relaxed.

2. Work on staying still—not a single muscle of the body should be moving. Only move an arm or finger once commanded, and choose which part of the arm or finger is going to move, when, how fast, and its final destination. Try practicing this with different parts of the body.

3. Try controlling the body's senses. Try practicing responding to a loud sound by moving only after you have analyzed the sound and have chosen when and how to move. There is no reason to move because of a loud noise from a scream when children are playing, a loud noise from an ambulance when not on the street, or a loud noise from music that is not going to harm you.

4. Try controlling the response to pain (e.g., if the knee hits a hard object, only respond when you have chosen to respond: screaming is not going to make the injury get better).

5. When someone surprises you at work, only move after you have determined who it is and how you are going to respond. Learn to control the senses by responding only after the mind has processed the initial sensation or stimulation, determined if it is worth responding to, and decided how to respond.

6. Try doing all these steps throughout the day; the longer you do them, the sooner you will see results. The body and organs need to adjust to your new mental processor, which controls the metabolism and autonomic body functions. This adjustment could take up to six months, depending on how well you can control the body's functions and how quickly you adjust to the new relaxed state of mind.

7. Try relaxing while driving. Try looking at all the cars as a whole rather than staring at every car at a fast pace while driving. Do not look at every individual inside every car while driving. Try relaxing while going to the mall. Try looking at all the individuals as a whole and not at each individual. The same advice applies to looking at the merchandise. Try looking at all the merchandise as a whole and not at each individual piece at a fast pace.

This reversal process helps an individual learn to control and stop the autonomic nervous stimulation that is making him or her age prematurely, feel more pain than he or she should, have allergies when he or she shouldn't, be hungry when he or she shouldn't be, lose his hair when he shouldn't, have attention deficit hyperactivity disorder when he or she shouldn't, have Parkinson's when he or she shouldn't, have

Alzheimer's when he or she shouldn't, or have excessive sexual desires when he or she shouldn't.

Detailed Steps to Reverse AHS in Six Months

Class – For an eighteen-year-old male
During the first month, practice the following techniques two hours a day, plus controlled movements throughout the day.

1. During the first month, try to learn to control the blinking of the eyes by staring at an object. Blink in a controlled manner, and blink by gradually moving the eyelids down and up. Try doing this on and off throughout the day.
2. Try controlling the speed of the eye movement while changing from staring at one object to another. Only move the eyes by choice. Try moving the eyes slowly from one object to another. Trying doing this on and off throughout the day until this technique is mastered.
3. Perform both of these eye exercises until you gain full control of the eyes. Learn to blink the eyelids and move the eyes slowly only when commanded.
4. Practice these exercises on and off throughout the day to increase effectiveness.

During the second month, practice the following techniques two hours a day, plus controlled movements throughout the day.

1. During the second month, try to clear the mind of all thoughts; try keeping the mind thinking of only one thought at a time.
2. Try slowing down the thoughts to a snail's pace, with

the goal of sounding slow or extremely calm to an outsider.

3. Try slowing down and controlling every movement of every muscle to the point where every muscle moves by conscious choice, and the speed and destination of each muscle movement is considered.
4. Practice these exercises on and off throughout the day to increase control and effectiveness.

During the third six-month period, practice the following techniques two hours a day, plus controlled body movement throughout the day.

1. Try eliminating harmful external motivations—TV, radio, commercials, intense movies, aggressive driving, and hyperactive work environments.
2. Try slowing down or relaxing the brain while jogging, running, or performing exercises over a long period.

Exercise versus No Exercise

Exercise can play a major role in reversing AHS if it is performed properly, but it could be counterproductive if it is done improperly or abused. Exercise exhausts the inner energy, which allows the mind to exert less of an effort to regain control of body movements.

Exercise with a slow mind to condition the mind to regain control of body movements over the autonomic nervous system. Exercise is used to develop the body's inner energy, strength, and endurance. The body's inner energy can be counterproductive, since the inner energy can be transformed into a destructive nervous energy or mental heat that can destroy the hair follicles.

Two systems control body movement simultaneously: the mind and the autonomic nervous system. They coexist to protect the body; one acts during an emergency or emotional condition, such as a competition when there is a need for a rush of energy, and the other takes control of the situation when there is a need for mind control. Exercise with a focus on slowing down the mind, even while running at top speed, to condition the mind to control body movements in order to reach maximum speed.

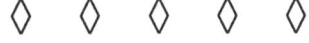

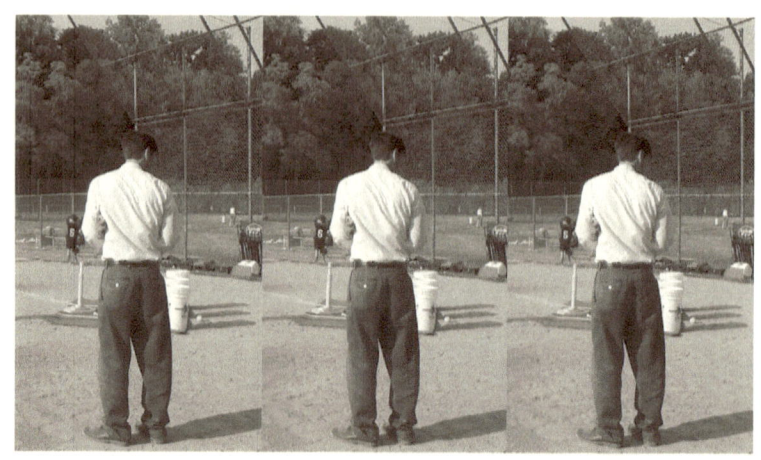

Chapter 13
Evolution of a Theory

Evolution of a Theory

Thirty-eight years ago, I was confronted with two paths in life; one path was to try to slow down to reduce stress, and the second path was to try to speed up to reduce stress. Both paths felt comfortable and natural and made me feel good, so it was difficult to choose. When my mind was relaxed, it felt happy, good, and energetic. When my mind was hyperactive, it felt full of energy and rushed, and it seemed like there was not enough time in the day to do everything. My mind was too busy to know how it felt. I chose the path to slow down, emulating the behavior of past generations. This seemed natural based on lessons learned from recent history and my own experiences. This choice became a hypothesis; it could be either true or false, or a little seed that could be either real or false. The hypothesis became a shift in paradigm or, as I saw it, a change in societal patterns, patterns that were not apparent or readily visible to an observer. The hypothesis started to grow and evolved over time; it became more complicated and developed into many concepts that needed to be confirmed as being true or false through observation and in-depth research. Observations and analysis led to findings over time; the hypothesis was confirmed to be true time after time.

The initial hypothesis evolved into a greater and more complicated problem. The little seed grew into a great tree, and it provided fruits for new discoveries. The search to understand how a seed grew to form a tree led to new revelations and at the same time provided a confirmation that the little seed was real after all.

Disproving the Theory

Over the last thirty-eight years, I have been trying to analyze and find situations where these engineering theories were true or false, learning more about baldness and its association with hyperactivity. The following questions were asked:

1. Why do some men not lose their hair?
2. Why do some overweight individuals tend to keep their hair?
3. Why do women keep their hair?
4. Why do tall individuals tend to keep their hair?
5. Why do smaller individuals lose their hair faster?
6. Why do older individuals tend to keep their hair?

All these questions were initially mysteries until the numbers started to follow distribution and grouping patterns. For instance:

1. Some of the men who were initially not bald started to become bald.
2. Some of the men who appeared to be out of the norm were actually wearing wigs.
3. The distribution of men with hair versus men without hair was changing.
4. Older men who traditionally kept their hair were also becoming bald.
5. Taller men who traditionally kept their hair were also becoming bald.
6. Foreign men who traditionally kept their hair were also getting bald.
7. Younger men who used to have long hair have chosen short hair.
8. Younger men who traditionally kept their hair were also becoming bald.
9. Women's hair that used to stay healthy was drying up and becoming thinner.
10. Men and women who would have typically had young hair in their forties were now getting white hair in their thirties
11. Overweight individuals who had typically kept their hair were also becoming bald.

Many of these changes were attributed to the work and external media environment. The intensity and demands of the workplace have increased over the last fifteen years. Changes occurred in the work environment where typically relaxing jobs demanded computer abilities, and even homes without any kind of external media coverage in foreign countries or homes in poor areas were also becoming statistics because of the exposure to satellite networks. Therefore, exposure to a fast or accelerated environment, whether at home or work, directly impacts the body's nervous system in most individuals, young or old, men or women, tall or small, overweight or skinny, but the extent of the impact is also related the body's ability to unconsciously learn new behaviors or a new accelerated state of mind.

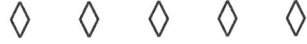

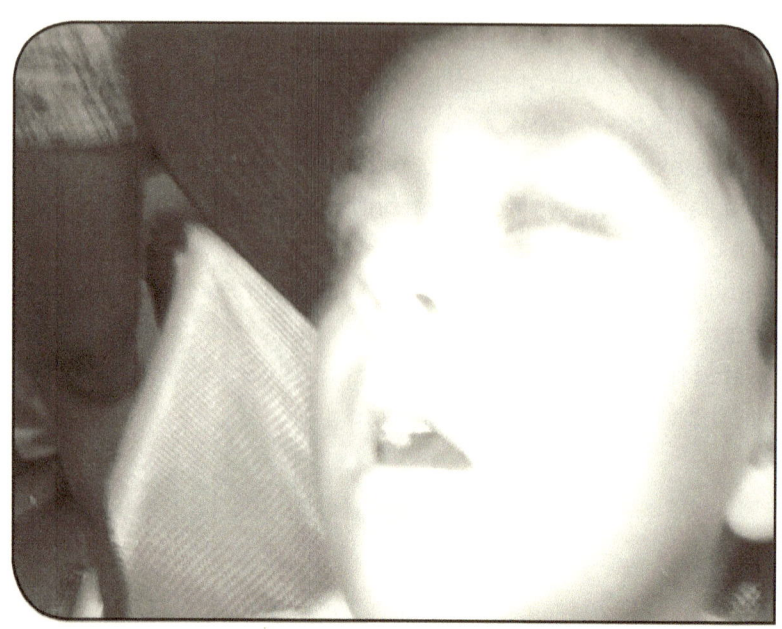

Chapter 14
The Mind Control Theory

What Is Mind Control?

This refers to the frontal part of the brain that controls the autonomic mechanism or the nervous mechanism of the brain. This is the system that we need to recondition or develop in order to regain control of the nervous mechanism or the nervous trigger.

What Is the Autonomic Mechanism?

This is referred to here as the nervous mechanism; it is located on the lower part of the brain or upper part of the spinal cord and contains and turns on the nervous trigger in response to a vigorous, panic-inducing, or emergency condition. The nervous energy needed by the autonomic mechanism is generated and supplied by the stomach.

What Is a Mind at Peace?

A mind at peace means a state in which AHS is no longer present, when there is a constant state of happiness without the need for material things or continuous food gratification. This is a state when boredom is no longer frustrating but satisfying, a state when the autonomic nervous system is no longer active and all body movements are under mind control. The nervous trigger has been turned off.

Loss of Values

Adapted AHS can reveal itself in a loss of family values. This means that the onset of AHS changes life as we know it. Life becomes urgency, where everything needs to happen quickly. There is a continuous need for food and material things; self-control or control of the body senses is impaired, which results in the loss of family values. This accelerated state causes side effects, such as hair loss, weight gain, wrinkles, gray hair, premature puberty, loss of looks early, or even early loss of mental acuity. This accelerated state of mind changes life and family values.

This accelerated condition alters the mind and changes our family values and the rules that were established or set up by previous generations. The mind changes to adapt to the accelerated pace, which causes our behavior to change. This change does not fit the norm, since it differs from the behavior and rules set by previous generations or our parents. This pace causes the body to actually mutate at an accelerated pace.

Specifically, these changes cause traditional rules of dating to become too old-fashioned; there is a need for rushed gratification, driving fast, impatience, and continuous food consumption because of the constant mental stress or uncontrolled autonomic nervous energy; thus, the pace of life appears to be too boring. Traditional rules established by previous generations no longer apply to children, teens, and young adults, middle-aged or even old individuals. Traditional rules of life are seen as outdated.

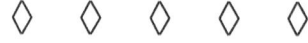

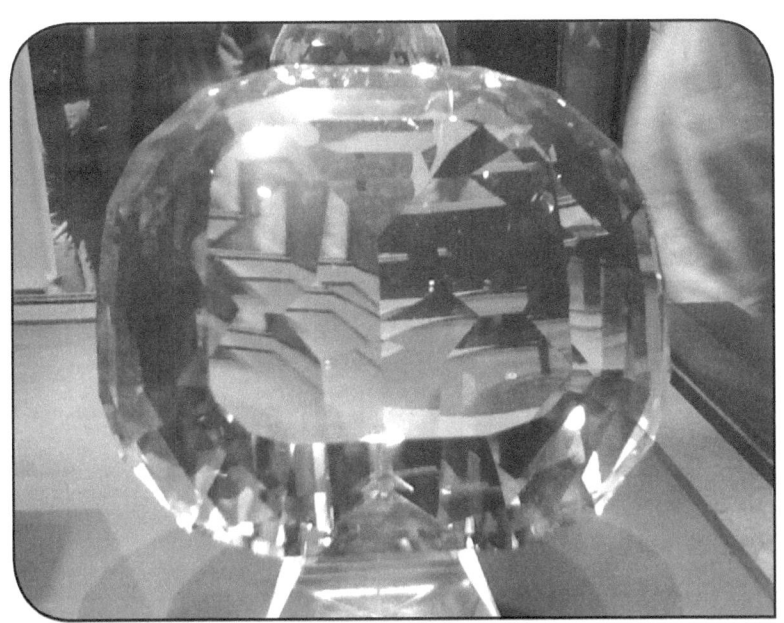

Chapter 15
Effect on Creativity Theory

Effects on Creativity

AHS reduces creativity because of the mind's inability to relax, explore the senses, and access stored memories. The accelerated operating frequency of the brain prevents the mind from retrieving memories that were stored at the body's lower natural frequency. AHS reduces the mind's ability to use the senses needed to observe, analyze, or create new ventures.

Creative Intelligence

Creativity or inventive intelligence can be reduced by AHS by preventing the brain from accessing or making the necessary connections. A brain that is overly stressed or utilized for useless information can become overloaded and function inefficiently. Avoid too much information, external media, video games, and Internet browsing. Again, expose the brain only to those things that are worth listening to and learning. As a rule of thumb, believe only 50 percent of what you see or hear and only 10 percent of what you read.

Brain Memory Storage/Retrieval Frequency Changes

Retrieving the Memory

The body's nervous system uses the body's natural frequency to store memories and thoughts, and then it uses the same frequency to retrieve the thoughts or stored memories. AHS increases the natural operating frequency of the mind either temporarily or permanently until the mind can no longer find or retrieve memories stored at the natural frequency. The connection between the mind and memories can be reestablished once the body's original frequency is restored.

Memory Blackout

A memory blackout is when the mind temporarily loses the ability to retrieve memories. This type of condition may occur during an exam, panic state, or an intense presentation. This condition occurs when the frequency of the mind (at the AHS or nervous condition) does not match the frequency at which the original memories were stored (at the natural or calm condition).

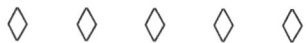

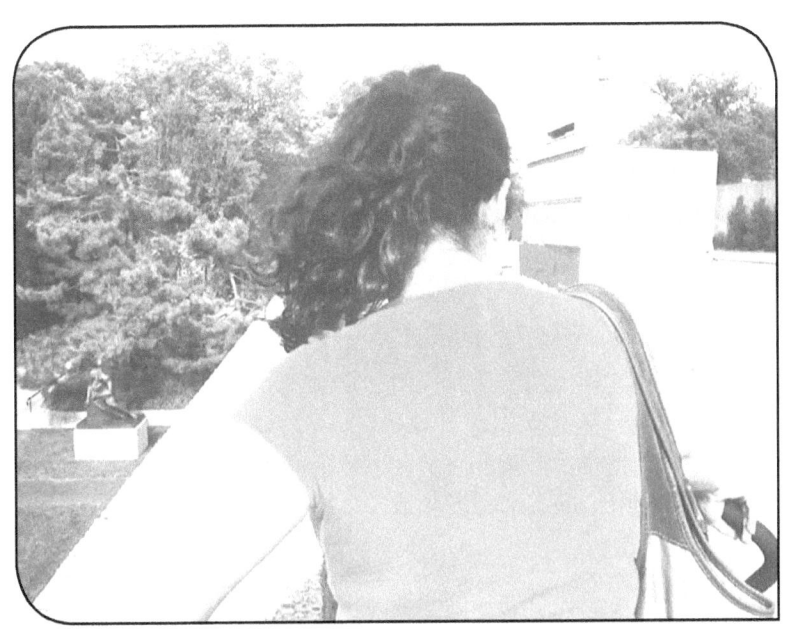

Chapter 16
Senses Control Theory

Effects on Increased Senses and Desires

AHS causes an uncontrollable need for gratification of the senses to satisfy intense urges and desires. Everything needs to happen more quickly; the clock has been accelerated, and anything other than superfast causes mental tension. AHS causes the body to move at an accelerated pace, resulting in accelerated aging, so everything needs to happen quickly before the clock runs out or the effects of aging set in.

AHS Effects Sexual Desires

AHS can lead to strong sexual desires, which results in oversexed behavior. There is a need for continuous sexual gratification. This excessive sexual activity can further accelerate the onset of AHS in a man, which results in rapid hair loss. This is more prevalent in men than in women. Stay away from all types of sexual activity, such as explicit adult magazines, go-go bars, adult Internet sites, and adult movies. Because the body adapts in as little as six months, this excessive sexual activity can be reversed and controlled in as little as six months to a year by applying controlled meditation techniques.

Allergies

High frequencies from TV commercials, fast movies, or computer use in the environment cause hyperactivity, which makes the nerves more sensitive. This hyperactive condition causes the body to be more sensitive to bacteria and foreign objects, which otherwise the body would have ignored. This sensitivity increases as an individual gets older, exercises less, and performs fewer outdoor activities. Exercise, if performed with a relaxed mind, can be a form of meditation; if conducted regularly, it can reduce or make the nerves less sensitive. Reducing the sensitivity of the nerves can prevent the outbreak of allergies.

Eye Movement

Exposure to the high frequency or flickering speed from TV commercials, movies, computers, and the environment causes the onset of hyperactivity, which makes the nerves more sensitive. Highly sensitive nerves intensify the vision (or intensify the images received), which causes the eyes to be more sensitive to light and causes them to become irritated; the eyelids then continuously blink to cool the eyes. Over time, repetitive blinking and excessive eye movements cause the formation of dark circles under the eyes.

AHS Effects on Vision

AHS could lead to overly sensitive eyes, resulting in excessive eye strain, which could lead to deformation or a change of the eye shape that could cause the early loss of perfect twenty-twenty vision.

Tiredness and Eye Tension

Most of the time, excessive eye irritation can be mistaken for the need to go to sleep, which in fact may be a form of stress. Sleeping under these conditions could be counterproductive and can cause additional stress instead of a good night's sleep. Sleeping while under stress may be harmful to the body and may lead to more stress, heart attacks, or stroke and more tiredness or lack of sleep. Instead of resting while under stress, perform light exercise as a means of releasing the stress. Slow down the mind first, and then proceed to get a good night's sleep. Perform light exercise for half an hour or more, depending on how long it takes you to feel comfortable. This light activity will release the stress, enabling you to sleep better and wake up rested without extending the amount of sleeping time.

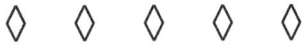

Chapter 17
AHS Effect on Global Warming

AHS Effect on Global Warming

AHS affects global warming. Accelerated and uncontrolled human behavior makes the human body produce more heat, have a tendency to be constantly rushed, work faster, drive faster, work longer hours, eat more food, burn more calories, need more toys, want bigger houses, want bigger cars, and so on. This statistical trend where a majority of individuals want more affects our planet. This chronic uncontrollable behavior can exceed the planet's ability to recuperate until all its resources are exhausted and humankind is driven to extinction. This accelerated pace can harm the planet's balance or life cycle. AHS is the cause or source of all these side effects, as shown in the following chart.

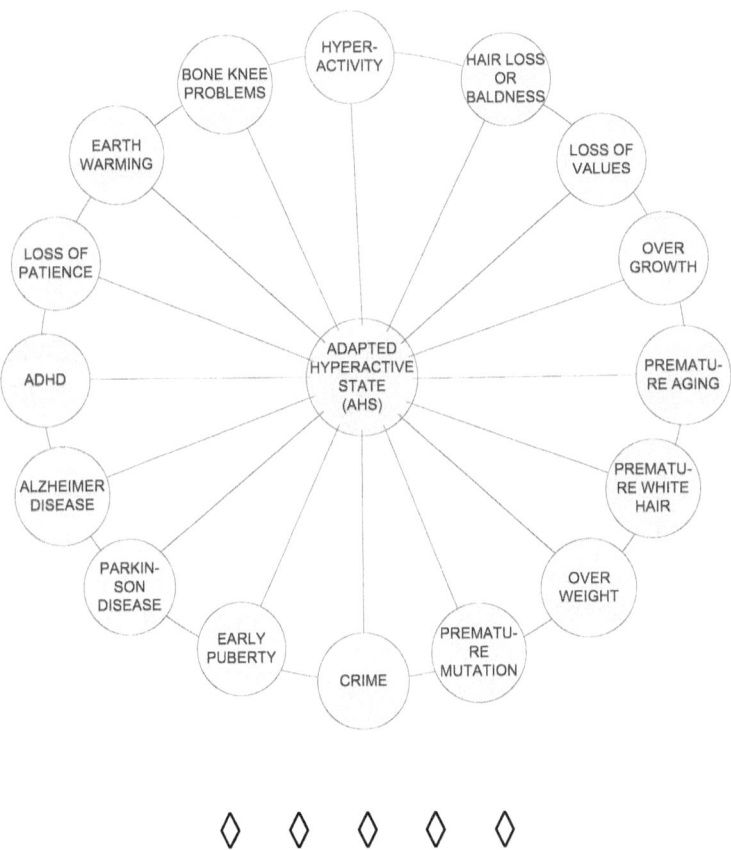

◊　◊　◊　◊　◊

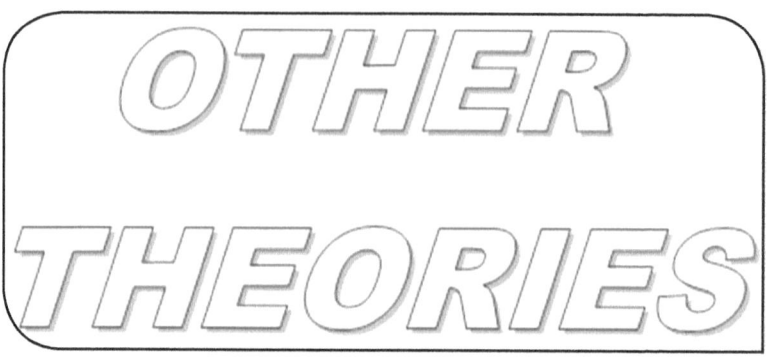

Chapter 18
Other Theories

Heart Attacks

Contrary to the current belief that heart attacks are hereditary or evolve slowly from a long history of heart problems, a heart attack can occur as soon as one day after improper eating or a high-cholesterol meal (pizza, ice cream, and eggs) combined with high stress. Heart attacks usually occur late at night or early in the morning, when the mental stress level is at the highest and there is a high demand for blood supply from the heart. This condition, along with the lack of physical activity, causes the cholesterol not to get properly processed, which results in additional accumulation of plaque in the arteries around the heart. The accumulation of cholesterol along with the high blood demand can cause the heart to get exhausted, falter, or stop working.

There are usually symptoms to help one recognize the beginning of a heart condition, such as body discomfort, high mental stress, tiredness, burning of the eyes, mild chest pain, or pressure around the heart area. To quickly counter this situation, an individual needs to reduce the body's mental energy demand while reducing the cholesterol concentration around the heart. To counter this condition, perform light heart compression-decompression exercises. These types of exercises can include light, side-to-side lateral torso flexing exercises at night to compress/decompress the heart and clear concentrations of cholesterol around the heart and arteries while reducing the body's stress level or mental energy demand. Perform at least five hundred repetitions of these exercises, or continue until the discomfort around the heart goes away and the body's stress level returns to a normal level. A high stress level can be detected by noticing eye irritations or the inability to go to sleep.

Resistance Theory

Take proper caution before giving a sick and fragile elderly person a tranquilizer to calm him or her down and make him or her feel better. The body's nervous or autonomic system operates by sending signals to the different parts of the body, including the heart to make it beat. A tranquilizer works by adding additional resistance to the nerve signals coming from the brain to reduce their intensity and calm the person's nerves. Giving a tranquilizer to an older person who already sends weak nerve signals to the heart can weaken the signal further and cause the heart stop. Giving a tranquilizer to an old or weak person is like giving him or her poison.

Explaining Migraines

Migraine headaches are caused by a temporary abnormal state of mind that occurs when the hyperactive nervous system of the brain is temporarily connected with the mind control system. Mind control accelerates to access data stored at the nervous frequency while trying to slow down and maintain control of body functions. For example, if an individual is hyperactive, this state occurs when he or she starts to slow down the temporary connection between the accelerated mind control, and the hyperactive nervous system causes a migraine until the mind loses control and the connection is lost. If an individual is a relaxed individual, this state occurs when he or she is exposed to a stressful or accelerated condition (e.g., a presentation, an emergency, or a panic-causing condition), the temporary connection between the mind control and the hyperactive nervous system triggers a migraine until the body relaxes once again.

Migraines Caused by Infections

Migraine headaches are also caused by minor infections in the body. Minor infections result in the accumulation of liquid in the brain when the body tries to fight the infection, which causes a congested head and can trigger a migraine.

Stomach Effects on the Immune System

The effectiveness of the immune system begins with how the stomach processes food. Keep the stomach healthy to strengthen the immune system. Alcohol weakens the stomach's walls and the immune system. Stress can affect the stomach's ability to function properly, and it weakens the immune system.

Excessive Alcohol

Excessive alcohol steals away the water from the body and therefore weakens the joints and muscles, which leads to cramps, pulled muscles, and joint pain. Continuous use of alcohol weakens the body joints, which can lead to premature cartilage damage and can cause permanent knee or joint damage. Alcohol removes the water from the joints, which takes away their flexibility and can increase rupture or wear.

Drinking alcohol weakens the walls and processing power of the urinary track system. Prolonged and repetitive exposure to alcohol weakens the organs' walls, their defense mechanism, and their ability to perform their functions.

Prevent Cancer

Since the stomach produces the body's immune system, it can fight the onset of cancer. A healthy stomach supplies healthy white cells to the blood that provide an immune system that kills cancer. Stress can affect the stomach and weaken the immune system.

The effectiveness of the immune system begins with how the stomach processes food. Keep the stomach healthy to prevent the onset of cancer. The stomach is the source of energy of the nervous system. The stomach is the battery or energy that energizes the nervous system. A healthy stomach leads to a healthy body.

Starve Cancer

Starve cancer of its vital nutrients to weaken its bite. Deprive cancer of beef and other meat products. Strengthen the immune system to overpower cancer.

Cancer

A hyperactive nervous state can cause the body cells to be in a constant state of change, which causes them to mutate. This hyperactive condition, along with the weakening of the immune system, can cause the immune system to fail to locate, identify, destroy, or prevent the formation of cancer cells in the body. Reversing AHS or reducing the stress level, along with a healthy and powerful immune system, helps the body's immune cells locate and kill cancer cells.

Strokes

Decongestants can cause strokes. Decongestants can increase the chances of having a stroke, especially as an individual gets older and his or her mind is operating at a higher mental intensity level. Reduce the intake of decongestants to reduce the chances of having a stroke. Do not take decongestants for several consecutive days. AHS, along with age, can intensify the effects of a decongestant, which could lead to a stroke.

Knee and Hip Joints

Stress can degrade hip and knee joints from infrequent exercise or use. Stress or adapted AHS can put additional nervous tension on knee and body joints to the point that it can weaken them. Stress along with continuous AHS results in the lack of energy to exercise, which weakens and softens joints and cartilage, making them susceptible to wear and tear and causing irreversible harm.

Sitting down for long periods of time in front of a computer while working in a stressful environment weakens the cartilage and joints, especially those of less-active individuals, such as many middle-aged or older individuals. Simple movements of the knees, such as getting up or just walking, can cause tears or excessive wear on an already weakened or soft cartilage. Cartilage damage can cause the knee to swell up, creating further damage. A damaged cartilage can take up to six months to a year to heal. Get up regularly, walk around, and exercise every other day to keep the joints flexible and strong, especially if the workday includes sitting down for most of the day.

Cartilage behaves like muscles and follows the same principle: if an individual does not use it, he or she loses it. Cartilage weakened by a lack of activity or exercise can lead to severe cartilage or bone damage at the joint. Cartilage has blood vessels, and they can heal from simple walking (no heavy impact). If an individual has a swollen knee, then he or she needs to move slowly until the liquid dissipates; this prevents further cartilage damage. Additional damage to already damaged cartilage takes longer to heal the second time around.

Lack of Exercise

Cartilage gets soft from lack of use. It is like muscle; it needs to be flexed to become strong and flexible enough to withstand the body weight or forces on the joint. Joint exercises are required regularly or at least every other day to keep cartilage flexible and healthy.

Gradually work to strengthen cartilage to a working

level. Cartilage needs to be strong enough to withstand and support the body weight. If cartilage is too weak, it tends to tear with simple movements, which causes the joints to swell up and eventually deteriorate. Strengthen the cartilage by strengthening the muscles around the cartilage. Perform light isometric exercises by stiffening the leg muscles or by pressing the leg against a hard surface without bending the knee. The intent is to compress/decompresses the cartilage without bending the knee. Perform repetitive muscle-strengthening exercises daily until the cartilage is strong enough to support the body weight. Perform only those exercises that do not cause pain at the joint. The main purpose of these exercises is to strengthen the muscles around the cartilage area, since strong muscles will help remove the forces that can injure the joint.

Flexing the cartilage makes it stronger. Isometric exercises can help strengthen the cartilage without causing damage. Perform isometric exercises that do not cause pain until the cartilage is strong enough to support the body's weight.

Flexing the bones makes them stronger. Flexing the bones makes them stronger by increasing the bone wall thickness. Exercise causes the bones to flex. Bones behave just like muscles and cartilage; they need exercise as frequently as every other day. Lack of exercise beyond two days causes the bones to decrease in strength.

Understanding Back Pain

Generally, individuals over thirty tend to become less physically active. This inactivity can weaken the back muscles and cause wear on the meniscus padding or disks located between the vertebrae. Weakened muscles cause the disks to support most of the bending forces, especially the disks located in the lower back or the lumbar area. This area of the back carries most of the body weight, and even minor bending efforts can cause the disk to slip out of place or move toward the back side of the vertebrae. Sometimes a movement or dislocation of as little as one eighth of an inch can cause severe back pain and discomfort and can lead to further disk damage. Fortunately, ruptured disks do heal because they have blood vessels around their perimeter; unfortunately, they may take a long time to heal—from three months to a year, if properly cared for.

Twisted Back

Do not try to straighten the back if there is a pinch on the disk. This advice is based on a basic engineering concept of weight versus rotational friction. Instead, have someone pull the weight axially upward to remove the load from the vertebrae or disk while trying to rotate or straighten the back. After the weight or load from the lumbar has been removed, the back can easily rotate around the injured area without causing pain or further damage. This process prevents additional injury and can restore the back into the proper position. Try keeping the upper body weight off the injured disk in order to prevent further damage.

Swelling Back

Once an individual has a slipped disk or if a disk has been out of place for a long time, a day or longer, some muscle swelling will develop around the disk area. This swelling prevents or makes it more difficult to get the disk back into its original position, since the swelling has displaced or filled in the void or space where the disk used to be. To determine if the disk has slipped toward the front or toward the back side of the vertebrae, perform the following test: If an individual has pain while bending down, then the disk slipped toward the back, and if an individual has pain while bending the back backward, then the disk slipped toward the front of the vertebrae. If the disk is displaced toward the back side of the vertebrae, tie a belt around the waist, and while placing the hand between the belt and the injured area on the back, put pressure or push the disk back into position. Hold the applied pressure for a long time or ten minutes or more a few times a day until the disk moves back and displaces the fluids that cause swelling.

A similar principle can be applied if the disk is displaced toward the front of the vertebrae. In this case, while leaning on the back, lift one knee and then both knees while putting pressure on the stomach. The lifting of the knees stretches the back while the stomach pressure tries to push the slipped disk toward the back and into position. An X-ray of the vertebrae can help an individual determine in which direction the disk has been displaced. Once the disk is back in position, keep the back straight and minimize rotation for a couple of days until the swelling goes down. Be sure to keep the back in a vertical position to promote fluid drainage down and away from the injured area, which may cause additional or permanent damage to the nerves and medulla. Body mobility allows the fluids to dissipate, which prevents further damage and promotes healing.

Bones

Bones generally get weaker or the wall thickness gets thinner when an individual stops exercising. Bones, like muscle, get thicker and stronger when they are flexed while exercising. Although bones do not flex as much as a muscle, they do flex when exercising. Jumping exercises or low-impact exercises cause slight flexing of the bones and make them stronger.

Types of Headaches

There are commonly two types of headaches, a congestive headache and a stress headache. The congestive headache is caused by a congested head or a head full of liquid under pressure, while the stress headache is caused by stress or nerves. The stress headache causes sharp, localized head pain. To determine which type of headache an individual may be suffering from, move the head from side to side; if pain is experienced while moving the head, then it is a congestive headache. Use ibuprofen-based medications, such as Motrin®, to reduce the swelling and pressure. Acetaminophen, aspirin, and caffeine tablets, such as Excedrin®, can work well to reduce stress headaches. I generally take Excedrin® with food to increase its effectiveness and to minimize the possibility of getting an upset stomach.

Congestive headaches are generally caused by an infection or a virus, while stress headaches are generally caused by the mind going in and out of a stressful situation.

Consuming Alcohol

After consuming alcohol, it is a good idea to drink lots of water to reduce hangover headaches and minimize damage to internal organs, especially the urinary track system. The more water an individual drinks, the lower the concentration of alcohol that passes though the body's digestive system.

The water dilutes and reduces the concentration of alcohol that stays in the body organs and minimizes organ damage. As a rule, drink a least one full glass of water for every small drink—the more water, the better. Keep a log of the name and year of alcoholic drink being consumed; some drinks may be more harmful than others, based on their ingredients and how they were processed, even in small quantities.

Acid in the Stomach

Acid can cause irreparable damage to the stomach. Acid in the stomach can be caused by a nervous state of mind. Do not allow the acid to stay in the stomach for any period of time; try to get rid of the acid immediately to prevent an ulcer or tissue damage to the stomach walls. If in pain, dilute the acid by drinking excessive amounts of water until the pain stops. An individual may need to drink four or five bottles of water or even more, depending on the pain. Repeat as necessary.

Cold

People, in general, are always exposed to cold or flu germs. Generally, a cold develops when the body is too weak or if it has acquired enough germs to exceed the body's immune system's fighting capacity. If the immune system is weak, the body is more easily prone to become ill from cold germs, even if there are only a small amount of germs in the body. If the immune system is strong, it takes a greater amount of germs to overcome it. A cold or flu virus can usually harvest itself easier when the body is in a stressed condition or when the immune system is weak.

Cholesterol

The body needs sugar and air to process protein that is necessary to proper functioning. When the body is not functioning properly or the digestive system is out of balance, these ingredients are not processed properly, which causes excessive bad cholesterol and fat to accumulate in the body. Changes in the work environment, such as getting or losing a job or even retirement, can cause a sudden change or reduction in activity, which can have a major impact on the body's stress level and proper functioning in a relatively short period of time, in as little as six months, especially at an older age.

Individuals, forty and older, have a greater risk of accumulating cholesterol from a sudden change in conditions. In order to combat this condition, staying active is critical. A daily routine, such as exercising during lunchtime, walking around the neighborhood, or getting up and moving around the hallway every one to two hours during a busy workday, is suggested.

Organs

When an individual exercises, the organs also exercise, making them stronger and reducing the chance of the person contracting a disease. Exercise causes the body to expel the bacteria or toxic material that otherwise would accumulate and cause the insides of the organs to sag and form deposits that can cause an infection or a disease.

Deep-Organ Massage

Pain and pressure in the lower organs can be immediately

relived by using the fingers to apply deep massage right to the affected organ. Lie down on a bed, and place a belt around the waist. Use your fingers to apply repetitive pressure into the stomach while pushing against the belt. Repeat this process for a hundred or more times until gases are released. While in a horizontal position, apply fast, repetitive depressions against the stomach or directly into the affected organs to press or squeeze out a blockage or gasses, clear an infection, or move fluids within the organ. Do not apply pressure if it causes sharp pain.

Go as deep as necessary, and move the fingers in and out (and up and down) in a fast, repetitive motion to cause the contents, blockage, gases, infections, or acid inside the organ or organs that are causing the pain to dissipate, dilute, or pass through. Continue to do this three times per day for a week or so, depending on the severity, until the pain stops. This process can get rid of the pain, swelling, or the beginning of a serious problem in as little as five or ten minutes per session. Once the blockage has passed through, the organ becomes softer. These massages should be applied gradually to prevent internal damage and allow the blockage to dissipate.

Getting Older and Gaining Wisdom

As an individual gets older, wisdom increases only if he or she is a good listener. Remember only those things worth remembering, filter out those things that do not make sense. Learn by listening to everyone. Everyone has something valuable to add to the complex puzzle called life that may be worth remembering.

Continuous Learning by Listening

A good listener is an individual who has the patience to listen to anyone—those who are well educated as well as those who are not, young or old—and also has the ability to filter out those items that are worth remembering or useful from all the information obtained or received during conversations. A person can collect enormous wisdom from friends or colleagues or receive that which has been passed down from older generations. A good listener needs to know what to retain and what to erase or forget.

Worries

Worries that last for a long period of time—two weeks or longer—can be devastating to the immune system of the human body. Worry weakens the body's defenses against diseases and handicaps the normal operation of the nervous system to the point that it can lead to body damage, such as cancer, hair loss, sickness, and weight gain. Happiness is a counter to worries. Try to keep the mind continuously busy doing fun projects or hobbies so that there is no room left for worries.

Side Effects of Infection

An infection can lead to other infections. An infection can cause the immune system to concentrate on one infected area, leaving other areas vulnerable to other diseases. It can steer the immune system away from fighting other diseases, such as a cold, flu, other infections, or a more serious illness. It can also trigger other infections; if the immune system is weakened by fighting an infection or virus, then other germs or viruses that otherwise would not have surfaced or would have been mitigated at the early stages can surface as an infection. These can be a skin infection or a more serious internal infection. Other triggered side effects can mask or hide a real infection.

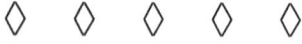

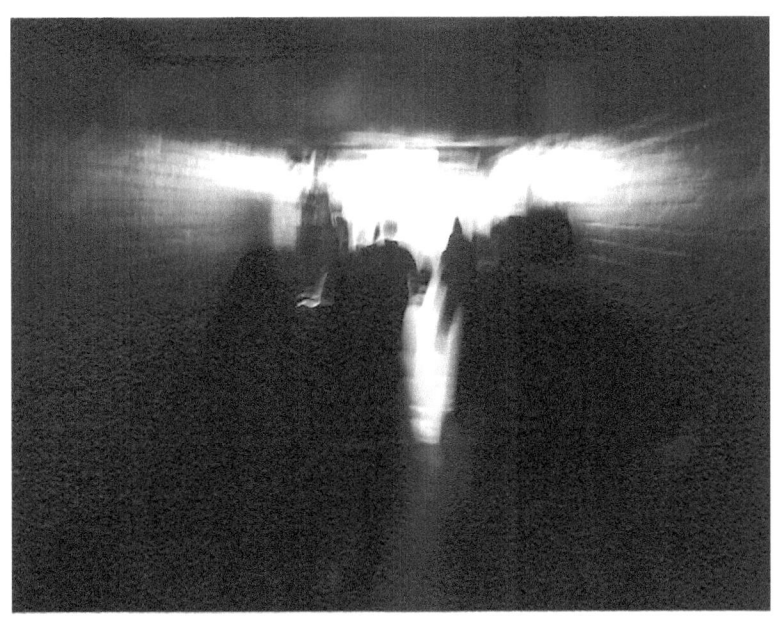

Chapter 19
Journey of the Mind

Journey of the Mind

Throughout most of the early part of my life, I was caught in an uncontrollable state of mind, but by mere luck, sacrifices, and making the right choices, I was able to find my way back to a peaceful and happy state of mind. Here is my journey to happiness.

I will take you on a journey to find yourself and the true meaning of happiness. So put all other worries and problems aside for now and learn to rediscover yourself. Where are you right now, and where are you going from here? You will discover the answer to these questions during the journey.

The Journey

It is not normal for an individual to be in an uncontrollable or rushed state of mind. The normal state of mind should generally be stable, controllable, happy, and relaxed.

The mind learns by doing and adapts to any state it is exposed to for a long enough period of time. This state could be a stress condition, nervousness, hyperactivity, calmness, happiness, frustration, or worry.

To adapt to a state means that the mind treats this new condition as the normal, every day and every night—even when you think you are relaxed.

Adaptation to a hyper state of mind can start in as little as two weeks, and adaptation can occur in six months when one is exposed to the hyperactive condition continuously for about eight hours per day (more or less depending on the individual). Initially, the mind flips back and forth from one condition to the other, prompting migraines, until it stays permanently in the hyperactive state.

Keep in mind that a relaxed mind can generally withstand numerous short periods of stress with no harm or side effects and return to normal (e.g., a fire drill on the job).

Once the mind adapts to a stressed condition, it takes as much time as one was in the stressed state, meditating to return to the normal state.

Once the mind is in the stressed state, if subjected to short periods of meditation, it will not return to a relaxed state. It takes extensive, repetitive meditation efforts to adapt and return the mind to the relaxed state.

The mind in the stressed condition causes the body to experience side effects.

The mind in the stressed condition does not rest or sleep. Nights are generally exhausting.

The mind in the stressed condition consumes its inner energy faster than it can generate it. This condition causes the body to deplete its inner energy prematurely or to lack energy.

The mind in the stressed condition forces the body organs to overwork and could cause harmful side effects, such as causing the body to generate excessive amounts of cholesterol, undergo premature aging, or suffer organ damage.

The stressed condition is not easily seen or felt. The body adapts to this condition in a form that may feel natural to the individual. Only the symptoms are observable.

The stressed condition causes hair loss but stops as soon as an individual reverses the process. The stressed condition causes the brain to work hard, creating extra heat in the scalp and promoting hair loss.

The stressed condition causes frustration, an upset state, and pain; promotes hunger; and exaggerates the body's feelings and senses. Stress amplifies the body's needs and causes weight gain. Eating provides temporary comfort.

The stressed condition could be hereditary, getting passed on in the genes.

Hereditary stress can be reversed but takes more time and effort.

Once an individual succeeds in returning the mind to its normal state, the hair starts to rejuvenate, grow, and become more flexible and healthier over a short period of time. All other side effects disappear.

Prolonged and repetitive exposure to the following conditions or factors could lead to a hyperactive condition:

⋄ fast-paced/high-stress job—constant pressure, too many meetings, trips, emails, problems, and so on
⋄ fast-paced computer work

⋄ fast-paced lifestyle
⋄ too many fast-paced commercials and television shows
⋄ excessive high-speed driving / traffic
⋄ constant worries
⋄ constant fear
⋄ too much caffeine
⋄ hereditary condition from a stressed parent

Remedies

1. You need to find yourself and learn to slow down. Find a place of total tranquility and where you can find peace of mind.
2. Try to be happy at all times.
3. Reduce fire drills on the job. Reduce the pace.
4. Do slow exercises. Once the mind is exhausted, it is easier to control.
5. You may experience migraine headaches during the transition from a stressed to a relaxed stage.
6. Once you find yourself, you need to maintain that relaxed state for a long enough period of time for the mind to adapt (six months or more).
7. Once the mind has adapted to the relaxed state, it is easier to control it, maintain the peace, and know when the mind is under stress.
8. Be yourself; be happy.

Everyone is different. Remember that each individual is unique. Since everyone is different, results vary. Individuals can be different in the following ways:

1. Some individuals have slow metabolism.
2. Some individuals have fast metabolism.
3. Some individuals have quick reflexes.

4. Some individuals have slow reflexes.
5. Some individuals are very smart.
6. Some individuals are not so smart.
7. Some individuals are very active.
8. Some individuals are not very active.
9. Individuals have different levels of hormones.
10. Women are different from men.
11. Men have high energy for short periods of time.
12. Women have low energy for long periods of time.
13. Some individuals are slow thinkers.
14. Some individuals are fast thinkers.
15. Some individuals are taller.
16. Some individuals are shorter.

Since everyone is different, there is the probability that each individual has proportionally different sized organs, which process things differently (i.e., for every action an individual does, there is probably a different output). Therefore, since everyone is different, each person should adjust the remedy and needs accordingly.

We humans used to be slaves to tradition, but we have lost our values and families in a world rushed by the media and computers. Now let's ask ourselves, what has changed?

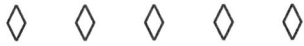

Index